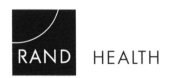

T0146263

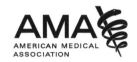

Effects of Health Care Payment Models on Physician Practice in the United States

FOLLOW-UP STUDY

RAND CORPORATION
Mark W. Friedberg, Peggy G. Chen, Molly Simmons,
Tisamarie Sherry, Peter Mendel, Laura Raaen,
Jamie Ryan, Patrick Orr

AMERICAN MEDICAL ASSOCIATION
Carol Vargo, Lindsey Carlasare, Christopher Botts,
Kathleen Blake

Sponsored by the American Medical Association

For more information on this publication, visit www.rand.org/t/RR2667

Published by the RAND Corporation, Santa Monica, Calif.

© Copyright 2018 RAND Corporation

RAND® is a registered trademark.

Cover image: freshidea / Adobe Stock

Support RAND
Make a tax-deductible charitable contribution at
www.rand.org/giving/contribute

www.rand.org

Preface

In 2014, RAND and the American Medical Association (AMA) conducted a qualitative research project entitled "Effects of Health Care Payment Models on Physician Practice in the United States" that described how alternative payment models such as capitation, episode-based and bundled payment, shared savings, and pay for performance affected multiple aspects of physician practice. Since 2014, alternative payment models have expanded to include new private, state, and federal programs—most notably the Medicare Access and CHIP Reauthorization Act of 2015 (MACRA) Quality Payment Program.

The project we report on here updates our 2014 study with qualitative data from physician practice leaders, frontline physicians, and other observers in the same six markets we examined in 2014. Whenever possible, we re-interviewed the same individuals who participated in the 2014 study. This allowed us to describe how their experiences with preexisting and new alternative payment models had evolved over a four-year period.

The current project began on October 18, 2017, and was completed on October 24, 2018. Project findings are intended to help guide efforts by the AMA and other stakeholders to improve current and future alternative payment programs and help physician practices succeed in a more value-driven environment.

This work was sponsored by the AMA. The opinions expressed in this report are those of the authors and cannot be interpreted as AMA policy. The research was conducted by RAND Health, a division of the RAND Corporation. A profile of RAND Health, abstracts of publications, and ordering information can be found at www.rand.org/health.

Table of Contents

Tables

Summary

Purpose

In 2014, RAND and the American Medical Association (AMA) conducted a qualitative research project entitled "Effects of Health Care Payment Models on Physician Practice in the United States" that described how alternative payment models such as capitation, episode-based and bundled payment, shared savings, and pay for performance affected multiple aspects of physician practice. This report updates our 2014 study with data from interviewees in the same six markets we examined in 2014. Our interviews focused on changes since 2014, including but not limited to the effects of new alternative payment models (APMs) such as the Medicare Access and CHIP Reauthorization Act of 2015 (MACRA) Quality Payment Program (QPP). Project findings are intended to help guide efforts by the AMA and other stakeholders to improve current and future alternative payment models and help physician practices succeed in them.

Methods

To describe the evolution of payment models and their longitudinal effects on physician practices since 2014, this project used the same qualitative multiple–case study method as our 2014 study, relying primarily on semistructured interviews with physician practice leaders, frontline physicians, and other observers. Whenever possible, we sought to interview the same individuals and organizational representatives that we interviewed in 2014. We then supplemented the sample with new interviewees, aiming to collect data on payment models and practices that have emerged since 2014. As in our 2014 study, we included a relatively large number of cases (31 physician practices in six markets) because we wanted to capture a diversity of practice sizes, specialties, and ownership models. To collect updated data on market context, we also interviewed market observers from the same categories we used in 2014: leaders of health plans and hospitals operating in the market, state or county medical societies, and state Medical Group Management Association chapters. The project did not seek to describe effects of alternative payment models on patient outcomes or the costs of care.

Main Findings

Persistent Findings: Challenges Associated with Alternative Payment Models

Our 2014 study identified several key challenges facing physician practices that participated in APMs. At the practice level, alternative payment models increased the importance of data and data analysis (as well as data deficiencies and inaccuracies). At times, alternative payment models also conflicted with each other and with government regulations, complicating practices' ability to respond in a constructive manner. For individual physicians, core clinical activities were unchanged, but participation in alternative payment models had increased the volume of nonclinical activities, particularly documentation needs. Finally, our 2014 study identified problems with data integrity and timeliness, errors in payment model execution (including inaccurate measure specification and patient attribution), incomprehensible incentives, and concerns about measure validity, all of which limited the effectiveness of alternative payment models.

All the challenges described by respondents in 2014 persisted in the current study. In particular, issues related to data continued to constrain practices' ability to understand and improve their performance. Operational errors in payment models also continued to be a source of frustration for physician practices, at times with financial consequences. In some cases, these negative experiences reduced practices' future willingness to participate in alternative payment models, even when offered by different payers. Because physician practices typically participated in multiple payment models from a variety of payers, challenges related to interactions between payment models also persisted.

Persistent Findings: Physician Practice Strategies Regarding Alternative Payment Models

As in 2014, practice leaders and other stakeholders across the study markets implemented a variety of strategies in response to APMs. These included new capabilities and models of care, investments in data and analytics, and internal financial and nonfinancial incentives for individual physicians. Some of these strategies were a continuation of previous efforts (e.g., expanding the roles of care management and care coordination staff), while others involved adding new capabilities (e.g., enhancing a primary care practice's ability to provide behavioral health services), often enabled by new information technology. Practices also augmented their capabilities to collect and manage data from internal and external sources by investing in staff and information technology.

Despite engagement with new APMs, most practices reported that internal financial incentives for individual physicians had not substantially changed since 2014. Modest bonuses for quality performance remained common, and with the exception of small, independent practices (for which physician-owner incentives were inseparable from practice-level incentives), individual physician financial incentives based on costs of care were almost nonexistent. As in 2014, practice leaders deployed a range of nonfinancial strategies to influence physician decisionmaking, such as internal performance reports, that appealed to physicians' competitiveness and self-esteem.

New Findings: Accelerating Pace of Change in Payment Models

Across study markets, multiple practice leaders and market-context interviewees perceived an accelerating pace of change in payment models since 2014. This acceleration, partially driven by the MACRA QPP, capped an already fast-paced prior decade of successive payment and regulatory changes including the Physician Quality Reporting System (PQRS), the Health Information Technology for Economic and Clinical Health (HITECH) Act, the Patient Protection and Affordable Care Act (ACA), patient-centered medical homes (PCMHs), accountable care organization (ACOs), and other pay for performance (PFP), shared savings, and episode-based payment programs. The pace of change was challenging for most practices and especially so for small and independent practices. Larger organizations described partially shielding their physicians from payment changes by focusing on long-standing internal goals and by modifying their internal incentives more slowly than the external incentives received from payers.

Market observers noted that practice management consultants were sometimes unable to keep up with the pace of change, making it harder for small primary care practices to find trustworthy advice. Some practice leaders called for a "time out" from further payment changes, so that they could better understand how to respond to their current financial incentives.

Sudden or unexpected discontinuations of APMs were particularly challenging for physician practices and other market participants. Respondents in the current study described these APM reversals as resulting from transitions in state and federal political leadership rather than the performance of the models themselves. In some cases, reversals undermined practices' ability to receive a return on their investments in performance improvement. In other cases, such as unanticipated shifts from APMs back toward FFS (fee-for-service) payment, physicians described feeling frustrated by the return of volume-based incentives.

New Findings: Increasing Complexity of Payment Models

Interviewees from a wide range of practices, markets, and roles said that alternative payment models have become increasingly complex since 2014, citing an expanding number of performance measures, uncertainty concerning performance thresholds for penalties and rewards, and interactions between different payment models as sources of this complexity. The MACRA QPP was a key contributor to this complexity because it introduced new decision points for practices (e.g., the choice between the Merit-Based Incentive Payment System [MIPS] or an Advanced Alternative Payment Model [AAPM], or the choice of performance measures from a large menu). Practices of all sizes and specialties reported that understanding complex new payment models often entailed a significant resource investment, either to hire consultants or to build internal capabilities to analyze APMs. In our sample, larger practices and those affiliated with large health systems made these investments, while leaders of smaller, independent practices were more likely to express confusion and disengagement.

For practices that did invest in understanding APMs, the increased complexity of payment models presented new opportunities for financial success. Some of these practices found ways to receive more credit for their preexisting quality—without materially changing patient care—by enhancing their documentation and data abstraction practices, thoroughly coding risk adjustment diagnoses, actively managing patient attribution, or purposefully selecting their performance measures to maximize the likelihood of rewards.

New Findings: More Prominent Risk Aversion Among Physician Practices

Despite general enthusiasm for APMs that involved bonuses, interviewees in practices that spanned multiple specialties and markets reported a high degree of financial risk aversion, which influenced their decisions to engage in new payment models. Risk aversion was especially prominent among practices that had experienced losses in APMs or that were inexperienced in managing risk. These practices sought either to avoid downside risk or to off-load it to partners (e.g., hospitals and device manufacturers) whenever possible.

For smaller practices, taking on debt to finance infrastructure investments that were necessary to succeed in APMs represented another form of financial risk. These practices were attracted to APMs that offered subsidies for up-front infrastructure investments and to partners that provided such infrastructure at nominal cost, in exchange for a share of any bonuses received. Some larger practices—especially those with prior experience taking losses in APMs—renegotiated their contracts to shift more risk back to payers.

Implications

Simpler APMs Might Help Practices Focus on Improving Patient Care

The complexity of new APMs has confused some physician practice leaders, disengaged others, and induced a small set of practices to make substantial investments in understanding these APMs in detail. When practices do not understand APMs, they are unsure of whether to invest in care improvement, or how to do so in ways that will be financially rewarded or reimbursed. However, when practices have invested in understanding these APMs, they can find ways to earn bonuses and avoid penalties without necessarily changing patient care (e.g., through strategies that affect patient attribution), especially when practice leaders believe their quality is already high. Our findings suggest that the greater the complexity of APMs, the greater the potential financial return on practices' investments in understanding them. Simplifying APMs might help tip the balance back toward improving patient care as the preferred strategy for earning financial rewards.

Practices Would Benefit from a Stable, Predictable, Moderately Paced Pathway for APMs

The accelerating pace of change in APMs has exhausted not only physician practices but also the consultants advising them. Worse, unanticipated reversals in payment policies have prevented practices from recovering the costs and reaping the rewards of their substantial APM-driven investments in care improvement. A slower, more predictable pace of change in payment models seems likely to benefit practices, payers, and other stakeholders. Practices might consider negotiating longer-term contracts with payers, with built-in penalties for early unilateral termination of the model (or substantial deviation from the prespecified course of change). To insulate APMs from the vagaries of electoral politics, efforts that involve private-sector payers might prove more stable over time.

Practices Need New Capabilities and Timely Data to Succeed in APMs

As in 2014, many physician practices in our current study—especially small, independent practices—reported that they lacked the internal skills and experience necessary to perform well in APMs. Data management and analysis were seen as critical skills; yet, without timely, complete, and accurate performance data, even practices with well-developed data infrastructures were unable to assess their improvement efforts, make course corrections, or even know their positions relative to performance targets. Helping practices invest in these skill sets and supplying them with timely, understandable performance data will likely be a critical contributor to the ultimate success of many APMs. Conversely, payment models that are poorly executed (e.g., with serious, persistent operational errors) and unsupportive of physician practices could undermine future engagement in APMs and fail to improve patient care.

Reducing Practices' Access to Upside-Only APMs Risks Disengaging Them

In our current study, physician practices expressed increasing aversion to downside risk in APMs (regardless of APM complexity). With the exception of larger practices that had extensive experience in managed care, practices generally sought upside-only APMs. When faced with

APMs that featured downside risk, practices took steps to off-load this risk to partners. Given this risk aversion, and given the likelihood that practices will find ways to minimize downside risk in any event, payers should carefully weigh the anticipated advantages and disadvantages of mandating APMs with downside risk. In some cases, continuing to offer upside-only APMs or finding other ways to help practices manage downside risk (e.g., subsidizing up-front investments in new practice capabilities) might improve APM uptake—especially among practices with limited experience in risk contracts.

Designing APMs to Encourage Clinical Changes That Individual Physicians See as Valuable Might Improve Their Effectiveness

As in 2014, physicians were broadly supportive of APMs that enabled their practices to make noticeable improvements in patient care. In such cases, physicians reported intrinsic satisfaction with clinical improvements, sometimes even when these improvements did not result in financial bonuses. However, when APMs' principal impact on physicians was to create new documentation and reporting burdens—or there was no perceptible improvement in patient care—physicians generally reported disengagement and skepticism that anything had improved, even when they received bonuses. Co-designing APMs with practicing physicians and other leaders of their practices might help improve physician engagement and the chances that APMs will produce real improvements in patient care.

Acknowledgments

We gratefully acknowledge the invaluable time, expertise, and knowledge generously contributed by leaders and physicians in the physician practices, leaders of state and county medical societies, Medical Group Management Association chapters, health plans, and hospitals that participated in this study.

In addition, we gratefully acknowledge the following individuals who provided input into the contents of this report: Carol Kane, AMA; Apoorva Rama, AMA; Chau Pham, RAND; Lea Xenakis, RAND; Shawna Beck-Sullivan, RAND; Jodi Larkin, RAND; Libby May, RAND; Emily Chen, RAND; and Samuel Edwards, Oregon Health & Science University.

Abbreviations

AAPM	Advanced Alternative Payment Model
ACA	Patient Protection and Affordable Care Act
ACE	Acute Care Episode
ACO	accountable care organization
AMA	American Medical Association
APM	alternative payment model
AQC	Alternative Quality Contract
BCBS	Blue Cross Blue Shield
BPCI	Bundled Payments for Care Improvement
CJR	Comprehensive Care for Joint Replacement
CMMI	Center for Medicare and Medicaid Innovation
CMS	Centers for Medicare and Medicaid Services
CPC	Comprehensive Primary Care Initiative
DSRIP	Delivery System Reform Incentive Payment
EHR	electronic health record
FFS	fee-for-service
HCC	hierarchical condition category
HITECH	Health Information Technology for Economic and Clinical Health
HMO	health maintenance organization
HRRP	Hospital Readmissions Reduction Program
IPA	independent practice association
MACRA	Medicare Access and CHIP Reauthorization Act of 2015
MGMA	Medical Group Management Association
MIPS	Merit-Based Incentive Payment System
MSSP	Medicare Shared Savings Program
PCMH	patient-centered medical home
PCP	primary care physician

PFP	pay for performance
PGIP	Physician Group Incentive Program
PHO	physician hospital organization
PO	physician organization
PPO	preferred provider organization
PQRS	Physician Quality Reporting System
QPP	Quality Payment Program (a program resulting from MACRA)
RVU	relative value unit
SNF	skilled nursing facility
VBP	value-based payment

Introduction

In 2014, RAND and the American Medical Association (AMA) conducted a qualitative research project entitled "Effects of Health Care Payment Models on Physician Practice in the United States" that described how alternative payment models such as capitation, episode-based and bundled payment, shared savings, and pay for performance affected multiple aspects of physician practice (Friedberg, Chen, et al., 2015). In that project—hereafter referred to as "our 2014 study" because all data collection and analyses were performed in 2014—we interviewed physician practice leaders, frontline physicians, local medical society leaders, Medical Group Management Association (MGMA) leaders, hospital leaders, and health plan leaders in six markets throughout the country: Little Rock, Arkansas; Orange County, California; Miami, Florida; Boston, Massachusetts; Lansing, Michigan; and Greenville, South Carolina.

The project we report on here updates our 2014 study with data from interviewees in the same six markets we examined in 2014. Our interviews focused on changes since 2014, including but not limited to the effects of new alternative payment models (APMs) such as the Medicare Access and CHIP Reauthorization Act of 2015 (MACRA) Quality Payment Program (QPP). Whenever possible, we re-interviewed the same individuals who participated in the 2014 study. This allowed us to describe how their experiences with preexisting and new alternative payment models evolved over a four-year period.

The current project began on October 18, 2017, and was completed on October 24, 2018. Project findings are intended to help guide efforts by the AMA and other stakeholders to improve current and future APMs and help physician practices succeed in a more value-driven health care environment.

Organization of This Report

This report begins with an update of the literature since 2014 on how APMs have evolved and affected physician practices. Next, we present our study methods and an update on key characteristics of each of the six study markets.

Our main findings follow, in two sections. First, we present findings that have persisted since 2014, with one chapter on the challenges associated with APMs, and a second chapter on physician practice strategies regarding APMs. Next, we present new findings, with one chapter on the accelerating pace of change in payment models, a second chapter on the increasing complexity of payment models, and a third chapter on more prominent risk aversion among physician practices. Each of the three chapters presenting new findings includes challenges and practices' strategies for addressing them.

Finally, in the conclusion, we present implications for physician practices, payers, and other stakeholders.

Literature Update: Effects of Payment Models on Physician Practices

Overview

In this section, we summarize the published literature on each payment model and organizational model discussed in this report: capitation and global payments, episode-based and bundled payments, pay for performance (PFP), shared savings, retainer-based payment, medical homes, and accountable care organizations (ACOs). As in our 2014 study (Friedberg, Chen, et al., 2015), we focus on literature examining the following:

- prevalence: We include historical and current estimates of the prevalence of the payment model
- incentives and interventions to affect individual physician decisionmaking: We summarize relationships between how practices are paid (payment models) and how practices incentivize and influence their physicians internally
- organizational changes: We present relationships between practice participation in payment models and changes to practice size, ownership, and affiliation with other organizations
- impact on physicians: We review relationships between payment models and physician professional satisfaction, work quantity and content, and overall compensation.

In addition, we describe two major health policy shifts that have occurred since 2014, both of which are highly relevant to the evolution of alternative payment models: the implementation of the Patient Protection and Affordable Care Act (ACA) of 2010 and the MACRA QPP. We summarize the published literature describing how these policy changes influenced physician practices' adoption of alternative payment models.

This literature update does not include effects of APMs on the quality or costs of patient care. Although the effects of payment models on patient care are extremely important (and are the main outcomes in most APM evaluations), they are outside the scope of this report.

Payment Models Included in the Scan

As in our 2014 study, we reviewed three categories of payment models: "underlying" payment models that can exist alone, without other types of payment (i.e., fee-for-service [FFS], capitation, and episode-based or bundled payment); "supplementary" payment models that can coexist with one or more underlying payment models but cannot exist on their own (i.e., PFP and shared savings); and retainer-based payment models as a variant of capitation. In this section, we briefly define each of the payment models studied. A more detailed description and conceptual model of different types of payment models and how they interact is available in the report from our 2014 study (Friedberg, Chen, et al., 2015).

Core Payment Models
Fee for Service (FFS)

In FFS payment models, the practice receives a payment per unit of service provided. Practices collect payment on a rolling basis by billing for each service unit they provide to patients and then receiving reimbursement from payers. In principle, once services have been provided, the practice should know with certainty the amount of FFS payment it will receive.

Capitation

In capitation models—also termed "global payment"—the practice receives a payment per patient per time period. Attribution rules are needed to determine which patients are assigned to a particular practice and hence what that practice's total capitated payment will be. In practice, payers commonly attribute patients to the physician that the patient identifies as his or her primary care physician, but more complex attribution rules can be used (e.g., to a practice that provides the majority of a patient's services). Capitated payments may cover all health care services or only a subset, and they may be risk-adjusted for patient characteristics. In traditional capitation models, practices receive up-front payments at prespecified time intervals (e.g., monthly, yearly). Capitation exposes practices to financial risk because of variations in the cost of care. These contracts may offer varying degrees of risk-sharing to offset these variations and to insure practices against unexpectedly high costs of care.

Episode-Based and Bundled Payments

Episode-based and bundled payments define a particular "episode of care" as the basis of payment. An episode of care can be defined in many ways, but typically it covers a particular diagnosis or procedure, as well as all related services over a specified period of time. A common example is bundled payments for arthroplasty, which may cover the surgery, the associated inpatient stay, physician fees, post-acute care, and any other services required for a window of time following the surgery. As with capitated payment, episode-based payment exposes practices to variations in the cost of care and is thus intended to incentivize cost containment. Episode-based payment contracts may also include some degree of risk-sharing.

Supplementary Payment Models
Pay for Performance (PFP)

In PFP models, practices receive bonus payments for satisfying specified performance goals. Both the basis of payment and the rate can vary a great deal. PFP payments can be based on productivity measures, quality of care measures, cost, patient outcomes, or some combination thereof. Rather than rewarding practices for desired outcomes, PFP programs may instead penalize practices for undesirable outcomes (e.g., Centers for Medicare and Medicaid Services [CMS]'s Hospital Readmissions Reduction Program). Payments to an individual physician can be calculated either on the basis of his or her individual performance or on the performance of his or her practice or physician organization (PO) as a whole—in the latter case, PFP bonuses may be paid to the practice or PO, which in turn can decide how to distribute these payments to individual clinicians. PFP models can be added to any of three core payment models: FFS, capitation, or episode-based payment.

Shared Savings

In shared savings models, practices are reimbursed via FFS as they provide services, and then periodically these payments are reconciled against a cost benchmark. In one variant of shared savings—"virtual capitation"—the cost benchmark is based on the expected total costs of care for the practice's attributed patient population. At the end of the year, the practice receives a lump-sum bonus if costs are lower than the benchmark. In another variant of shared savings—"virtual episodes"—the cost benchmark is based on the expected cost of a particular episode of care. Episodes are identified retroactively at the end of the year, and practices receive a lump-sum bonus if their costs of care during these episodes are lower than the benchmark. In contrast to traditional capitation and episode-based payment models, in virtual capitation and virtual episode models, practices receive a *share* of the observed savings relative to the cost benchmark. All shared savings models incorporate upside risk in this manner; some, but not all, also incorporate downside risk, where practices pay a penalty if actual costs of care exceed the cost benchmark.

Retainer-Based Payment

Retainer-based payment models—also known as concierge or direct pay models[1]—require a supplementary capitation payment per patient per time period, also called a "membership fee." This fee allows a patient access to the practice, and it may cover a defined set of services separate from those services that are billed to the patient's insurance. Except in cases where the membership fee is intended to cover all primary care services that a health plan would typically cover, the fee must often be paid out-of-pocket. Finally, retainer-based payment models often reduce the overall number of patients seen in a practice.

Organizational Models That Combine Payment Models
Medical Homes

There are many different definitions of medical homes, but, in essence, practices designated as medical homes are expected to proactively manage patients' curative and preventive health care needs and coordinate any medical care they receive across different entities. To achieve these goals, many medical homes incorporate some form of case management services. The majority of medical homes are primary care practices, though, as described below, there are a growing number of specialty-based medical home models as well. Just as the features of medical homes vary, so do the models for paying them. While the most common revenue source is FFS, most medical homes are eligible for additional payments that may include enhanced FFS rates, per-patient per-month fees (i.e., care management or medical home fees), PFP, or shared savings arrangements.

Accountable Care Organizations

As with medical homes, there are numerous definitions of ACOs, as well as numerous payment models for ACOs. ACOs are broadly defined as health systems or collections of practices that jointly enter a contract with a payer to manage the health care needs of an attributed patient population while meeting quality and cost targets. ACOs are typically paid via either traditional capitation or virtual capitation models that incorporate PFP. Shared savings are typically paid as a lump sum at the end of the year, but other types of rewards are possible (e.g., enhanced FFS rates for the following year).

---

[1] "Concierge" models are a subset of "direct pay" models. The distinction is price, which is higher for concierge models than for other direct pay models.

Approach

We conducted a structured search of the peer-reviewed evidence regarding alternative payment models in the United States. To identify original research and review articles we searched PubMed, Business Source Complete, and EconLit for English-language articles published from 2014 through June 2018 (i.e., since our previous study). A complete list of search terms is included in the online Appendix. To identify additional grey literature on this topic, we searched LexisNexis and the New York Academy of Medicine Grey Literature Database: These searches were variations of those conducted in the bibliographic databases, adjusted as needed to fit the search capabilities of each. We focused on articles that specifically addressed the prevalence of alternative payment models and their effects on physicians' incentives, the structure of health care organizations, and physicians themselves (i.e., professional satisfaction, work content, compensation). We did not include literature examining the effects of alternative payment models on patient outcomes or the costs of care. Two researchers independently reviewed titles and abstracts to identify publications relevant to our study.

Value-Based Payment: Overall Landscape

There are roughly 950,000 licensed physicians in the United States, practicing in a variety of settings (Young et al., 2017). Based on data from 2016, 42.8 percent of U.S. physicians practice in single-specialty groups; 24.6 percent practice in multiple-specialty groups; 16.5 percent are in solo practices; 7.4 percent are employed directly by hospitals; 3.1 percent are in faculty practice plans; and 5.7 percent in other settings (Kane, 2017).

The most recent estimates of the prevalence of value-based payment (VBP) are derived from the 15th Annual Physician Practice Preference and Relocation Survey, a national survey of 2,219 physicians and advanced practice clinicians across different specialties conducted by the Medicus Firm, a physician search firm. As of May 2018, 43 percent of respondents were certain that their compensation plan included at least some value-based pay, up from 41 percent in 2017. Of these respondents, half reported that the value-based component amounted to less than 10 percent of their total income (The Medicus Firm, 2018). Further details on the prevalence of specific types of value-based payment models are described below.

Capitation

The report from our 2014 study includes a section on older capitation efforts, such as the managed care expansion of the 1990s (Friedberg, Chen, et al., 2015). Here, we review more recent literature on this topic.

Prevalence

While capitation is rarely used as the *sole* reimbursement model for physician practices or individual physicians—in 2013, for example, only 5.3 percent of physician office visits were covered under pure capitation arrangements (Zuvekas and Cohen, 2016)—capitated contracts commonly make up at least part of a practice's business. In 2015, 46 percent of primary care practices participated in at least one capitated contract (Levine, Linder, and Landon, 2018). Capitation is more common in the western United States (Zuvekas and Cohen, 2016). These findings from the published literature mirror the findings of our 2014 study.

Notable examples of capitated arrangements at the physician organization level among public payers include Medicare's Pioneer and Next Generation ACO models (note that capitation is optional under these models), Maryland's global budget program for hospitals (Edmondson, 2015), and Oregon's coordinated care organizations in Medicaid (Stecker, 2014; Angier et al., 2017). Among private payers, Blue Cross Blue Shield (BCBS) of Massachusetts's Alternative Quality Contract (AQC) remains one of the most extensively studied examples of providing global payments at the physician organization level (Song et al., 2014; Mechanic, 2016). Other well-known organizations participating in capitated arrangements with private payers include Intermountain (Bendix, 2015), Iora Health (James and Poulsen, 2016), and the California Public Employees' Retirement System (CalPERS) with Blue Shield (Chen and Fan, 2016).

The limited growth in capitation models has often been interpreted as evidence that they are unpopular among provider organizations, but low employer enthusiasm may be another growth-limiting factor. In Massachusetts, for example, the growth of global payment slowed between 2012 and 2015 as commercial plans decreased their risk-based, health maintenance organization (HMO) offerings and shifted more enrollees to FFS preferred provider organization (PPO) products including high-deductible plans (Mechanic, 2016).

Incentives and Interventions to Affect Individual Physician Decisionmaking

Under capitation and global payment models, organizations are no longer incentivized to increase the volume of visits: This has led some to argue that capitation may facilitate more fundamental delivery system shifts toward nonvisit care. Modeling the effects of capitation arrangements on practice revenues, however, suggests that capitation must make up the majority of practice revenues before there are sufficient incentives to move away from the traditional visit-based care model (Basu et al., 2017).

Related to this, a key concern about capitation arrangements has always been that they might incentivize "too little" care overall (Brosig-Koch et al., 2017). Physician organizations receiving capitation therefore tend to shield individual physicians from the incentive to reduce services—by paying them a salary or on an FFS basis (Allen-Dicker, Herzig, and Kerbel, 2015; James and Poulsen, 2016; Zuvekas and Cohen, 2016)—and incentivize quality improvements by adjusting payments to physicians on the basis of quality outcomes (James and Poulsen, 2016). This finding is unchanged since our 2014 study.

Since 2014, the published literature suggests that a growing number of organizations are adjusting payments to individual physicians on the basis of costs (James and Poulsen, 2016), or they are incentivizing cost containment through shared savings opportunities (e.g., giving physicians bonuses for cost containment) (Bendix, 2015; Mechanic, 2016).

Organizational Changes

Capitated payments may prompt physician organizations to be more cost conscious when developing external referral networks. Iora Health's strategy, for example, is to develop relationships with a narrow network of specialists whose practice style aligns with their philosophy (Bendix, 2015). Otherwise, we did not identify any literature examining how capitation has shifted organizational models.

Impact on Physicians

There is limited recent literature on the impact of capitation and global payment models on physician satisfaction, and most of what we found is largely drawn from the experience of specific institutions. Iora Health's founder, for example, reported that decreased time spent on billing and coding has enhanced physician satisfaction within the organization (Bendix, 2015). Physicians at the Beth Israel Deaconess Medical Center in Boston—an academic medical center—were surveyed four years after entering a global payment contract. The majority of physicians, 85 percent, were supportive of the model, citing perceived reductions in the cost of care and increased competitiveness in the health care market as the major reasons for their support (Allen-Dicker, Herzig, and Kerbel, 2015). The minority of physicians who were *not* supportive of the model cited concerns that it did not improve health care quality or physician satisfaction.

Episode-Based and Bundled Payments
Prevalence

Episode-based and bundled payment models have increased among both public and private payers since 2014. Medicare has taken an active role in this space. Below are some of the key Medicare bundled payment programs.

Acute Care Episode (ACE) Demonstration: Launched in 2009, this three-year voluntary demonstration piloted global payments covering Part A and Part B services for a set of inpatient cardiovascular and orthopedic procedures. Post-acute care was *not* considered part of the episode of care. Five hospitals located in Texas, Oklahoma, New Mexico, and Colorado participated (Urdapilleta et al., 2013).

Bundled Payments for Care Improvement (BPCI): In this voluntary demonstration launched in 2013, participants select one of four different payment models, each of which define an "episode" of care and organize reimbursement somewhat differently. Models 2 and 3, by far the most popular, include post-acute care and involve a retrospective bundled payment arrangement, in which providers receive FFS payments but total expenditures are reconciled against a target payment amount determined by CMS. During Phase 1 of BPCI—the "preparation" period—participants receive data from CMS to help prepare for possible implementation of bundled payments. During Phase 2—the "risk-bearing implementation" period—organizations become full participants and assume risk for medical expenditures (Centers for Medicare and Medicaid Services, 2016). The number of organizations joining BPCI has grown over time, though there has been significant attrition between Phases 1 and 2 (Evans, 2015a; Tsai et al., 2015). In the earlier years of BPCI, Model 2 participants that progressed to Phase 2 tended to be large, nonprofit academic hospitals in the northeastern United States, and these participants tended to enroll in bundles for a smaller subset of the eligible clinical conditions that were also higher volume (e.g., joint replacement, congestive heart failure, chronic obstructive pulmonary disease, and pneumonia) (Tsai et al., 2015). As of April 1, 2018, there are 1,100 BPCI participants: 273 acute care hospitals, 535 skilled nursing facilities (SNFs), 194 physician group practices, as well as home health agencies and inpatient rehabilitation facilities (Centers for Medicare and Medicaid Services, 2018a).

Comprehensive Care for Joint Replacement (CJR) Model: This mandatory bundled payment model for hip and knee replacement was launched in 67 geographic areas in 2016. As of February 1, 2018, approximately 465 hospitals were participating (Centers for Medicare and Medicaid Services, 2018a). This model includes a cap on financial risk for all participants, though the cap is more generous for rural and community hospitals (Wadhera, Yeh, and Joynt Maddox, 2018).

CMS's transition from voluntary to mandatory bundled payment models—including CJR and proposed mandatory bundled payments for cardiac care, initially planned for 2018—was initially viewed as a signal that episode-based payment was likely to become more widespread. In late 2017, however, CMS cancelled the mandatory cardiac bundles, prompting questions and uncertainty about the future of these models in Medicare (Wadhera, Yeh, and Joynt Maddox,

2018). At that time, CMS also changed the CJR model from mandatory to voluntary for rural and low volume providers and, in 33 of the 67 original geographic areas, made the program voluntary for *all* providers (Centers for Medicare and Medicaid Services, 2018b).

Among private payers, bundled payments are considered the fastest-growing form of value-based payment (VBP): Commercial health plans responding to McKesson Health Solutions's 2016 survey on VBP made 11 percent of their payments under bundles, and they expected that number to rise to 15 percent after two years, and to 17 percent after five years (Whitman, 2016a). Bundled payments have traditionally been used to finance surgeries and other procedures, and they have been particularly popular for joint replacements. A 2015 survey of members of the American Association of Hip and Knee Surgeons found that 46 percent were participating in bundled payment models (Lieberman, Molloy, and Springer, 2018). Bundles have also expanded into new clinical areas, such as maternity care (Whitman, 2016b) and cancer care (Herman, 2014).

Incentives and Interventions to Affect Individual Physician Decisionmaking

Physician organizations that participate in episode-based and bundled payment models are predominantly paid FFS up front: This finding is unchanged since our 2014 study. At the end of each year, total costs are reconciled against the cost benchmark for the episode/bundle, and any savings are returned to the organizations. Physician organizations may then distribute these gainsharing payments to the individual physicians performing the procedures (Althausen and Mead, 2016). In some cases, shared savings are also distributed to the hospitals hosting the procedures, and to other providers, such as visiting nurses (Whitcomb et al., 2015).

Organizations that participate in episode-based and bundled payment models have also used nonfinancial incentives to motivate their physicians to achieve higher quality care at lower cost. For example, some have found that allowing physicians to see how their cost and quality performance compares to that of their peers can motivate performance improvement (Meyer, 2017). This was also a finding in our 2014 study.

If payments are not appropriately risk-adjusted, there is a chance that episode-based and bundled payment models will exclude more medically complex patients, whose care may be costlier (Elbuluk and O'Neill, 2017; Courtney et al., 2018), or select performance metrics that are perceived to be more under clinicians' control (Althausen and Mead, 2016). The former possibility has raised concerns for providers and policymakers alike about whether bundled payment models may decrease access to care among patients with greater comorbidity (Humbyrd, 2018).

Organizational Changes

Several distinct organizational shifts in response to episode-based and bundled payments have been noted in the literature:

(1) standardization of care processes
(2) migration to lower-cost sites of care
(3) migration to higher-volume or more specialized providers
(4) increased collaboration between proceduralists and post-acute care.

Our 2014 study also identified standardization of care protocols as a key organizational change associated with bundled payments. The other three trends linked to episode-based and bundled payments were identified in the current study. Much of the literature detailing these changes is derived from the experience of orthopedic bundled payments, in particular arthroplasty, where bundled payments have been growing in popularity.

Standardization of care processes: Episode-based and bundled payments create an incentive to prevent postprocedural complications, since the cost of treating these complications is subtracted from the bundle. Many institutions have responded by creating more standardized "care pathways" that attempt to reduce the risk of complications through interventions at each stage of the care continuum. Preprocedurally, there has been a greater emphasis on the identification and optimization of medical comorbidities before proceeding to surgery (Bolz and Iorio, 2016; Gray et al., 2018). Periprocedurally, some institutions have strengthened infection control strategies, pain management, and anesthesia protocols, and they have emphasized early physical therapy and enhanced discharge planning (Gray et al., 2018). Postdischarge, many institutions have engaged care coordinators to communicate with patients and post-acute care facilities, and they have established guidelines for the outpatient management of minor complications to avoid unnecessary rehospitalization (Bolz and Iorio, 2016).

Migration to lower-cost sites of care: In recent years, there has been a growth in ambulatory surgical centers, where arthroplasty can be performed as a day surgery, coupled with affiliated "orthopedic care suites," where patients receive dedicated nursing care and physical therapy until they are able to be discharged home (Elbuluk and O'Neill, 2017). By avoiding inpatient hospitalization following surgery, and the associated overhead costs, it is estimated that the overall cost of the procedure can be reduced by as much as 30 percent (Elbuluk and O'Neill, 2017). Candidates for outpatient arthroplasty are limited to patients without significant comorbidities and with a low likelihood of complications from the procedure. As a result, case migration has been accompanied by more careful advance screening and risk-stratification of patients (Bolz and Iorio, 2016). Patients deemed too complex for outpatient surgery are referred to hospitals for their procedures (Elbuluk and O'Neill, 2017).

Migration to higher-volume or more specialized providers: Bundled payments may create an incentive to shift cases toward higher-volume, more specialized providers who tend to achieve greater quality at lower cost. In response to BPCI, one institution encouraged only high-volume joint surgeons to perform arthroplasty, and they encouraged only "traumatologists" to manage fractures (Althausen and Mead, 2016).

Increased collaboration between proceduralists and post-acute care: For bundled payments for procedures, the costs of rehabilitation and post-acute care are subtracted from the bundle, thus creating an incentive to minimize these costs. As a result, proceduralists report trying to discharge patients directly home whenever possible (Bolz and Iorio, 2016). But when post-acute care is necessary, much greater attention is paid to the quality and costs of care at rehabilitation facilities than was previously the case: One study found that skilled nursing facilities (SNFs) with higher star ratings were more likely to participate in BPCI (Cen, Temkin-Greener, and Li, 2018). Several hospitals report identifying "preferred rehab partners" to whom they preferentially discharge patients (Bolz and Iorio, 2016), and providers also report greater collaboration between proceduralists and post-acute care providers after discharge, with the goal of decreasing complications (Wadhera, Yeh, and Joynt Maddox, 2018).

Impact on Physicians

Few published studies have examined the impacts of episode-based and bundled payments on physician satisfaction, but those that have report generally positive findings. In a survey of members of the American Association of Hip and Knee Surgeons (AAHKS) in 2015, 61 percent of respondents reported that they were planning to participate in bundled payment models, and 45 percent believed bundles would improve quality and decrease costs of care (Kamath et al.,

2015). In successful bundled joint replacement programs, clinicians have expressed satisfaction that these models tend to foster greater collaboration, and they are pleased to see lower costs and improved patient health outcomes (Meyer, 2017).

While clinicians have generally expressed agreement and satisfaction with the quality improvement incentives that are embedded in bundled payment models, they have also expressed reservations about the incentives for case selection (Humbyrd, 2018). In the AAHKS survey cited above, 94 percent of respondents worried that bundled payments create disincentives to operate on high-risk patients (Kamath et al., 2015). Clinicians have expressed concerns about how shared savings and other performance incentives would be distributed when multiple providers and entities contribute to a patient's outcome (Kamath et al., 2015; Wolinsky, 2016); frustration with their diminished autonomy and ability to individualize patient care (Dickson, 2015); and concerns that many high-cost complications are related to patient health problems that are beyond their control (Elbuluk and O'Neill, 2017). Concerns about unanticipated, uncontrollable costs were similarly cited by respondents in our 2014 study who were participating in bundles.

As bundled payments expand to new clinical areas beyond surgeries and procedures—for example, congestive heart failure and cancer—concerns about uncontrollable variability in the costs of care have become more pronounced, and enthusiasm for the model has dampened (Meyer, 2018; Murciano-Goroff et al., 2018). Oncologists have questioned how bundles might account for the high cost associated with many novel medications used for cancer, and they have expressed concerns that strict cost limits might disincentivize the use of these agents, even where they have been shown to improve survival and the quality of life (Muldoon et al., 2018).

Pay for Performance
Prevalence
Pay for performance (PFP) remains widely used by public and commercial payers, both as a standalone VBP strategy and as a component of other payment and care delivery models such as capitation, ACOs, and PCMHs (patient-centered medical homes) (James and Poulsen, 2016). The most sweeping shift in the PFP landscape since 2014 is the adoption of the Merit-Based Incentive Payment System (MIPS) in Medicare, a result of the passage of MACRA. Quality reporting under MIPS began in 2017, and the first payment adjustments will occur in 2019. We discuss the literature on the MACRA QPP and its impact on physician organizations in greater detail below.

Other prominent examples of PFP in the public sphere include CMS's Hospital Value Based Purchasing (HVBP) Program (Joynt Maddox et al., 2017), CMS's Hospital Readmissions Reduction Program (HRRP) (Wasfy et al., 2017), and Medicaid waivers for Delivery System Reform Incentive Payment (DSRIP) (Gusmano and Thompson, 2015).

Incentives and Effects on Physician Decisionmaking
PFP programs reward practices and provider organizations for achieving desired outcomes—or, as is the case in the HRRP, they can penalize practices and provider organizations for achieving undesirable outcomes such as excess readmissions. Rewards and penalties may be based on a variety of performance areas including: quality of clinical care (Johnson et al., 2015), effective coordination with other providers and improved transitions of care (Tejedor-Sojo, Creek, and Leong, 2015; Kamermayer, Leasure, and Anderson, 2017), patient experience (Stanowski, Simpson, and White, 2015; Pines et al., 2018), and cost reduction (Zygourakis et al., 2017). It

has been proposed that PFP programs might also reward equity and reductions in disparities in health outcomes, though rewards specifically tied to disparity reduction are not widespread (Anderson et al., 2018).

PFP programs that reward organizations add further complexity to the incentives that individual clinicians face. Clinicians facing organization-level quality incentives do report some positive effects, such as greater collaboration with colleagues and decreased likelihood of shifting complex patients with poor outcomes to other providers. At the same time, however, organization-level incentives can decrease individual clinicians' sense of control over their performance bonuses, thus potentially creating resentment toward colleagues "free-riding" off of their higher-performing peers (Greene et al., 2015).

Clinicians and provider organizations have questioned whether performance improvements can be sustained after PFP incentives are removed (Benzer et al., 2014). Moreover, there are concerns that some PFP incentives may be blunted by other competing financial incentives, or that clinicians may respond to incentives in unintended and undesirable ways. As an example of the former, while the HRRP penalizes readmissions, it does not address the substantial incentives to admit and readmit patients in the first place under diagnosis-related group (DRG)-based reimbursement. An example of the latter would be an increased use of observation status and the emergency department as settings in which to manage patients who would otherwise be readmitted (Carey and Lin, 2015). The possibility that extrinsic financial incentives might erode clinicians' intrinsic motivation and altruism has also been suggested, though empirical evidence of this erosion in health care settings is scant (Himmelstein, Ariely, and Woolhandler, 2014; Janus, 2014).

Organizational Changes

PFP programs that reward or penalize outcomes that may not be entirely under an organization's control—such as hospital readmissions—have in some instances prompted increased coordination between hospitals and other organizations and providers that influence patient outcomes. In the case of the HRRP, for example, some hospitals have developed a preferred network of SNFs (McHugh et al., 2017), while others have engaged pharmacists to follow up with patients after discharge (Arnold et al., 2015).

Internally, physician organizations have employed a variety of strategies to earn performance bonuses, with care management being one notable example (Wiley et al., 2015). Similarly, our 2014 study found that practices increased the scope of activities of allied health professionals in order to achieve quality goals.

Impact on Physicians

Our 2014 study identified numerous frustrations with PFP: the multiplicity of incentives; lack of alignment of performance measures across payment programs; difficulties in capturing accurate performance data; documentation burden; doubts about the clinical validity of performance measures; and perceptions by practice managers and frontline clinicians that pressures to satisfy the measures could, at times, distract from improving the quality of care.

The recent literature shows that while many clinicians support the use of financial incentives to improve care delivery and quality in principle, many of the concerns identified in our prior study persist, and clinicians express reservations about whether PFP schemes as currently designed can achieve their goals (Harrison et al., 2016). The availability, accuracy, and timeliness of data to aid in quality improvement initiatives is cited as an important prerequisite for successful PFP programs, but this is an area where gaps are frequently observed (Alidina et al., 2014; Abrahamson et al., 2015; Hussain et al., 2016). Providers have also reported a number of concerns about potential unintended consequences of PFP, including possible harm to patients, overlooking patient values and preferences, narrow measures distracting clinicians from giving optimal overall care, frustration over both increased documentation requirements and a perception that documentation is emphasized over actually improving patient care, and decreased morale and resentment over which team members receive the incentive (Xu and Wells, 2016; Hysong et al., 2017). Finally, there are concerns that safety-net facilities may face particular challenges in satisfying performance metrics and may thus be disproportionately penalized under these programs, depleting their already limited resources (Bazzoli, Thompson, and Waters, 2018; Roberts, Zaslavsky, and McWilliams, 2018; Shakir, Armstrong, and Wasfy, 2018).

Shared Savings Programs/ACOs

As in our 2014 study, the literature on shared savings programs derives largely from studies of ACOs. Therefore, in this section we describe the impacts of shared savings in the context of ACOs, noting that ACOs may also blend elements of other payment models such as PFP.

Prevalence

In 2014, it was estimated that 20 percent of U.S. hospitals were participating in an ACO (Colla, Lewis, Tierney, et al., 2016). Early adopters tended to be large, academic and not-for-profit hospitals (Epstein et al., 2014). ACOs have increased in prevalence since that time, across both public and private payers (Barnes et al., 2014; Kessell et al., 2015). One survey showed that participation in Medicare ACOs had increased by 2 to 3 percentage points between 2014 and 2016 (Rama, 2017). Public ACO models include the Medicare Shared Savings Program (MSSP), the Comprehensive ESRD Care Initiative, the Pioneer ACO Model, and the Next Generation ACO Model, as well as a growing number of Medicaid ACOs in states such as Oregon and Massachusetts. As of January 2017, there were 562 Medicare ACOs, and it is estimated that 10.5 million Medicare beneficiaries have participated in an ACO since the program launched in 2012 (Schur and Sutton, 2017). In 2015, an estimated 44 percent of primary care practices were participating in an ACO (Levine, Linder, and Landon, 2018). Another survey showed that 44 percent of physicians were in practices participating in at least one type of ACO, with participation rates of nearly 21 percent for Medicaid ACOs and 32 percent for Medicare and commercial ACOs. In that study, participation was higher for physicians in multispecialty practices compared with those in solo or single-specialty practices (Rama, 2017).

Incentives and Effects on Physician Decisionmaking

There are two principal types of ACO models: one-sided risk and two-sided risk. In one-sided risk models, organizations share in any savings that accrue to the sponsoring payer; in two-sided risk models, organizations must also pay a percentage of any costs that exceed a predetermined cost benchmark. To date, one-sided risk models have been more popular among provider organizations (Castellucci, 2017a), but payers, including CMS, are increasingly asking ACOs to bear downside risk as well (Vaughn et al., 2016).

Several challenges in structuring organization-level incentives for ACOs have been highlighted in the literature. First, even in one-sided risk models, some health care leaders report that the cost of achieving the population health management goals stipulated by ACOs is considerable and that they are not always able to recoup this investment through shared savings (Chen, Ackerly, and Gottlieb, 2016). The challenge of making ACOs financially viable is evident in the Pioneer ACO program: Within its first two years, 41 percent of organizations exited, most citing problems with the program's incentive structure, cost benchmark, and risk adjustment methods (Perez, 2016). These challenges were also cited in our 2014 study.

Second, there are concerns about incentives to "game" the cost benchmark determination process and risk adjustment methods. For example, in MSSP, organizations' cost benchmarks were initially determined based on spending levels in the several years prior to joining an ACO, thereby creating an incentive for organizations to inflate costs just prior to implementation (Douven, McGuire, and McWilliams, 2015). In the case of the Next Generation ACO program, CMS reported that coding intensity among ACO participants had increased so dramatically that, to ensure the financial sustainability of the program, it would be necessary to adjust participants' hierarchical condition category (HCC)-calculated average risk scores downwards, thereby making it more difficult for participants to earn savings and bonuses under the program. This has frustrated physicians and practices who argue that the increased coding intensity reflects the actual complexity of their patient populations (Castellucci, 2018b).

Third, while physician practice-controlled ACOs have a clear incentive to reduce costly inpatient and emergency department care, hospital-controlled ACOs may face conflicting incentives between decreasing costly episodes of care and ensuring sufficient inpatient volume to keep hospitals viable (Blackstone and Fuhr, 2016). This conflict was also identified by respondents in our 2014 study.

The principal strategy through which ACOs "transmit" incentives for quality improvement from the organization level to participating physicians is via internal PFP schemes, in which physicians receive bonus payments as rewards for high performance (Addicott and Shortell, 2014). Performance incentives may be tied to individual or group performance (Addicott and Shortell, 2014). Bonuses are commonly tied to the quality performance of an ACO, with efforts being made to incentivize valuable clinical services rather than clinical volume alone (Hacker et al., 2014). Less frequently, bonuses for groups and individual physicians may be tied to an ACO's financial performance (Addicott and Shortell, 2014). As discussed below, a major emphasis of ACOs has been strengthening primary care. In the early years of MSSP, the largest share of incentives was distributed to primary care physicians (PCPs) (Evans, 2015b): PCPs received 49 percent of shared savings, specialists 11 percent, and hospitals 9 percent (Schulz, DeCamp, and Berkowitz, 2015).

A key challenge in "transmitting" incentives downstream to physicians is limited physician awareness and understanding of the performance incentives—this was noted in the literature on shared savings programs and ACOs. In a survey of more than 1,400 physicians participating in MSSP from 2014 to 2015, nearly half did not know if they were eligible for shared savings or if their organization faced any downside risk (Schur and Sutton, 2017). Many physicians also did not know which of their patients were attributed to ACOs (Schur and Sutton, 2017).

In addition to financial incentives, a number of ACOs have used nonfinancial incentives to motivate quality improvement and cost savings among physicians. Examples of such strategies include transparency of physicians' quality performance and peer comparisons (Addicott and Shortell, 2014). In some ACOs, physicians are also explicitly encouraged to refer patients primarily within the ACO (Addicott and Shortell, 2014). Both of these findings mirror our 2014 study.

Organizational Changes

The increasing consolidation of health care organizations and the acquisition of physician practices by hospitals began over a decade ago and has continued in recent years alongside VBP reforms (Neprash, Chernew, and McWilliams, 2017). While it has been hypothesized that the growth in ACOs may have accelerated consolidation, there is little evidence to indicate that ACOs themselves—versus broader health care market forces—are responsible for these trends (Cuccia, 2014; Leslie and Blau, 2014; Alpert, Hsi, and Jacobson, 2017; Neprash, Chernew, and McWilliams, 2017; Richards et al., 2018). In fact, there is anecdotal evidence that some small practices pursue ACO affiliation as a strategy to *avoid* being purchased by hospitals or health systems: These practices feel that ACOs provide many of the benefits of system affiliation, such as supporting performance improvement activities and sharing the administrative burdens of quality reporting and billing, while allowing them greater autonomy in managing the practice than would a hospital (Castellucci, 2018a; Terry, 2018).

It appears, however, that ACOs have promoted increased partnership and coordination across different health care delivery organizations. Whereas a key theme in our 2014 study was the impact of ACOs on relationships between individual physicians and their referral patterns, the focus in more recent literature is on changes in relationships between health care organizations in the ACO landscape. One recent study found that 81 percent of ACOs involved new partnerships between independent health care organizations. The motivations for forming such partnerships included resource complementarity and risk spreading (Lewis et al., 2017). In developing partnerships, ACOs have tended to emphasize building an affiliated primary care network, with less attention to engaging specialists or other types of health care delivery organizations, such as post-acute care or hospice (Kuramoto, 2014; Colla, Lewis, Berquist, et al., 2016; Driessen and West, 2017; Driessen and Zhang, 2017; Kim et al., 2017; McWilliams et al., 2017; Resnick et al., 2018). The majority of existing ACO partnerships are based on preexisting positive relationships, but a minority involve organizations that were previously in competition (Lewis et al., 2017). Indeed, a key tension for ACOs lies in the role of cooperation—versus competition—in achieving lower health care costs (Grogan, 2015), and a major unsettled question is whether ACOs could come under antitrust scrutiny if they result in decreased competition in local health care markets (Barr and Mattioli, 2014; Berenson, 2015; Feinstein, Kuhlmann, and Mucchetti, 2015; Foote and Varanini, 2015; Kleiner, Ludwinski, and White, 2016). Developing shared governance and accountability mechanisms across participating entities has also been a challenge for ACOs (Addicott and Shortell, 2014). Some ACOs serving more disadvantaged populations (e.g., the Minnesota Integrated Health Partnership, a Medicaid ACO) have contracted with providers of behavioral health and nonmedical services in recognition of the distinctive needs of disadvantaged populations (Blewett, Spencer, and Huckfeldt, 2017).

Internally, as in our 2014 study, key organizational priorities of ACOs have been transforming primary care practices (Harris, Elizondo, and Brown, 2016) and strengthening care management and the engagement of allied health professionals (Shortell et al., 2014; Baloh et al., 2015; Pittman and Forrest, 2015; D'Aunno et al., 2016). Other more recent internal organizational trends include developing clinical integration tools across partners (e.g., shared medical records) (Kim et al., 2017), improving care transitions (Hacker et al., 2014), and quality improvement activities (Balasubramanian et al., 2018). In the early phases of implementation, there has been relatively little emphasis on standardization of care delivery processes across practices (Lewis et al., 2016).

Impact on Physicians

Among VBP models, ACOs have been particularly effective in engaging physicians in leadership roles. The National Survey of ACOs, fielded from 2012 to 2013, found that 51 percent of ACOs were physician-led, and another 33 percent were led jointly by physicians and hospitals. Physicians constituted a majority of the governing board in 78 percent of ACOs, and 40 percent of ACOs were physician-owned (Colla et al., 2014).

Whether increased physician leadership has translated to greater engagement of frontline physicians in ACO delivery models is unclear. As discussed above, many frontline physicians participating in an ACO have limited awareness of the incentives they face (Schur and Sutton, 2017). Primary care physicians tend to be more knowledgeable and engaged with ACO activities than specialists, and primary care physicians may perceive that they stand to gain more financially from these models than specialists (Stock et al., 2016)—and, as the evidence described above suggests, this perception is well founded (Schulz, DeCamp, and Berkowitz, 2015).

Even when awareness of incentives exists, physicians' views of ACOs have been mixed. Many see a shift to more team-oriented care as a positive change, though not all feel that they have the skills to lead a multidisciplinary care team (Stock et al., 2016). A number of physicians have been frustrated by the lack of quality measure alignment between ACOs and the other payers with which they contract (Addicott and Shortell, 2014). While many primary care physicians report that ACOs' *stated* goals of improving population health and improving health care delivery systems align with their motivation for pursuing a career in medicine (Stock et al., 2016), not all are confident that ACOs—as currently designed—can achieve these goals. In a survey of physicians practicing in Medicare ACOs, for example, only half felt that ACOs were effective models for the delivery of high-quality, low-cost medical care (Schur and Sutton, 2017). Many of these sentiments are similar to those identified in our 2014 study.

Finally, a number of physicians have expressed anxiety about the impact that ACOs will have on their compensation, control, and autonomy (Stock et al., 2016). In a recent survey of 82 ACOs in MSSP Track 1, 71 percent of ACO leaders said they would likely leave MSSP if forced to accept more risk, citing concerns about unpredictable policy changes by CMS, and a desire for more predictable financial projections (Dickson, 2018b).

Retainer-Based Payment

Examples of retainer-based payment include concierge medicine and direct primary care (DPC). Compared to concierge practices, DPC practices tend to charge lower retainer fees and attract a more socioeconomically diverse patient population (Eskew and Klink, 2015; Huff, 2015).

Prevalence

Retainer-based payment models are not prevalent, but they are increasing in number (Colwell, 2016; Grant, 2016). A 2014 survey of members of the American College of Physicians found that only 1.3 percent identified themselves as participating in a retainer-based payment model (Doherty, 2015). A 2016 survey by the Physicians Foundation found that the share of physicians practicing some form of concierge medicine had increased to 7 percent, with nearly 10 percent of practice owners planning to convert to concierge medicine in the next one to three years (Livingston, 2017).

Growth in retainer-based payment has been observed mostly in smaller, stand-alone practices (Krivich, 2017). Retainer-based payment models originated in, and are still primarily concentrated in, primary care practices, but recently these models are being taken up by specialties where patients have a longitudinal relationship with physicians, such as cardiology and endocrinology (Beaulieu-Volk, 2015a). One barrier to the adoption of retainer-based models has been regulatory uncertainty about whether practices can accept payments from health savings accounts to finance retainer fees or participate in state-based insurance exchanges (Pofeldt, 2016).

Incentives and Effects on Physician Decisionmaking

In retainer-based payment models, physicians do not need to bill on the basis of the volume of visits. As a result, these models do not incentivize physicians to bring patients in for issues that can be resolved by other means or to see as many patients in as short a period of time as possible. Consequently, physicians report doing more virtual visits and maintaining a smaller panel size (Finkel, 2017). We did not identify any other published evidence on how practices with retainer-based payment models incentivize their physicians.

Organizational Changes

Some practices with a retainer-based payment model have been partnering with employers to offer primary care services to their workers (Johnson, 2015), and some organizations, such as General Motors, have even contracted directly with health systems to provide a wide range of health care services with payment based on quality and cost savings (Greene, 2018). In the General Motors model, there are also some features of more traditional primary-care focused retainer-based payment such as guaranteed fast (even same day) appointments (Reindl, 2018). A key finding in our 2014 study was that some practices converted to retainer-based payment models to escape the pressure to merge into larger systems. Aside from one study that found that DPC practices predominantly included four or fewer clinicians (Eskew and Klink, 2015), we found no other recent literature discussing the impact of retainer-based payment models on organizational changes.

Impact on Physicians

There is limited published evidence on the impact of retainer-based payment models on physician satisfaction. Anecdotally, physicians who participate in these models report being happy with the flexibility they afford—including the ability to spend more time with patients, the reduced time and effort devoted to billing, and their exemption from MIPS (Johnson, 2015; Finkel, 2017). Similar sentiments were observed in our 2014 study. Some, but not all, physicians report that participation in retainer-based payment models has increased their income (Johnson, 2015). Practices that rely on retainer-based payment models do not need to attract as large a patient volume as traditional practice models to cover overhead expenses, which some physicians report can be a source of worry (Beaulieu-Volk, 2015b; Pofeldt, 2016).

Patient-Centered Medical Homes
Prevalence

As of 2013, it was estimated that 18 percent of office-based PCPs worked in patient-centered medical homes (PCMHs) (Hing et al., 2017); by 2015, 41 percent of primary care practices identified as certified PCMHs (Levine, Linder, and Landon, 2018). PCMH initiatives supported by public payers include Medicare's Comprehensive Primary Care Initiative (CPC), Comprehensive Primary Care Plus (CPC+), the Federally Qualified Health Center (FQHC) Advanced Primary Care Practice Demonstration, and the Medicaid Health Homes State Option. In recent years, there has been a growth in private and multipayer PCMH initiatives as well (Carrillo et al., 2014; Friedberg, Schneider, et al., 2014; Cole et al., 2015; Takach et al., 2015; Sarinopoulos et al., 2017). The majority of PCMH models remain focused on primary care, but recently there has been more experimentation with "intensive medical homes" and "specialty medical homes" for patients with advanced chronic illness who require close follow-up by specialists (Walker, 2017).

Incentives and Effects on Physician Decisionmaking

As in our 2014 study, the dominant form of physician payment within PCMHs is FFS augmented by per member per month care management fees and PFP bonuses (Quinn, 2017). Nationwide surveys of PCMH initiatives indicate, however, that the size of these additional bonuses may be increasing and the use of shared savings models is gaining traction (Edwards, Bitton, et al., 2014). Initially, shared savings models in PCMHs featured only one-sided risk (Edwards, Abrams, et al., 2014). CPC classic and CareFirst Blue Cross Blue Shield's PCMH initiative are two prominent examples of PCMH models that incorporate shared savings (Afendulis et al., 2017). Frontline PCMH physicians, however, are not always aware of the financial incentives they face (Afendulis et al., 2017). Nonfinancial incentives used in PCMHs include reports on physicians' quality and spending patterns (Maeng et al., 2015).

Organizational Changes

Externally, PCMHs typically pursue less formal integration with other facilities, as compared to ACOs (Edwards, Abrams, et al., 2014). However, certain PCMHs have evolved toward a broader "medical neighborhood" structure in which they proactively identify and engage specialists, hospitals, skilled nursing facilities, and even pharmacy chains that frequently serve their patients, all with the goal of enhancing communication and coordination (Maeng et al., 2015; Albanese, Pignato, and Monte, 2017; Luder et al., 2018).

Internally, PCMHs have adopted a variety of organizational changes and delivery models. Two key features identified in our 2014 study that remain prevalent are greater use of care coordinators (Afendulis et al., 2017) and reorientation toward team-based care, in which physicians work more closely with allied health professionals to co-manage patients (Harrod et al., 2016; Hing et al., 2017; Wagner et al., 2017; Prudencio et al., 2018; Rogers et al., 2018). A study of CPC practices identified several other common organizational changes, including increased risk stratification of patients, to identify those in need of more resources, efforts to expand patients' access to the practice, and data-driven quality improvement initiatives (Peikes et al., 2018). As in our 2014 study, the costs of practice transformation remain considerable (da Graca et al., 2018): HealthTexas, for example, spent approximately $43,000 per practice to achieve initial NCQA Level III PCMH recognition—and they noted that any savings in medical expenditures as a result of these investments would be recouped by third-party payers, not the practices themselves (Fleming et al., 2017).

Impact on Physicians

Physicians' experiences with PCMH transformation, as reported in the literature, have generally been positive: 96 percent of practices participating in CPC are continuing to the model's next phase, CPC+ (Dickson, 2017). When interviewed about their experiences, most PCMH practice managers in Minnesota were supportive of the medical home model and reported that they would adopt it again (Fontaine et al., 2015). Physicians also expressed appreciation for the additional care coordination support included in some PCMH models (Afendulis et al., 2017; O'Malley et al., 2017; Okunogbe et al., 2018).

However, a number of practices have reported that current financial incentives embedded in PCMHs do not go far enough to encourage practice transformation. Some practices have advocated for multipayer medical home models extending beyond Medicare to create stronger incentives for change (Dickson 2017). Others have argued that FFS-based reimbursement, which remains prevalent in PCMH models, is a barrier to delivery system change and that global payments would better align with the model's goals (Fontaine et al., 2015).

Practice leaders who expressed frustration with PCMH initiatives noted that not all payers provide adequate per member per month care management fees, that electronic health records (EHRs) often are not designed to support the goals and activities of the PCMH, and that PCMH participation is often associated with an increased burden of quality measurement and reporting (Fontaine et al., 2015; Peikes et al., 2018). Also, while the PCMH emphasis on interprofessional team-based care is generally appreciated (Wan et al., 2018), many practices—of physicians and allied health professionals alike—report uncertainty about how to function optimally as a team, define roles and distribute tasks, and take on additional work (Ferrante et al., 2018; Fiscella and McDaniel, 2018; Goldman et al., 2018).

Policy Changes

The Affordable Care Act

Since our 2014 study, there have been numerous shifts in the health policy environment that could potentially influence the adoption of APMs. The first is substantial changes to the Affordable Care Act (ACA). Late 2013 marked the opening of the health insurance exchanges, and in 2014 the individual mandate to have health insurance went into effect. As of January 1, 2014, 25 states had adopted the Medicaid expansion, and since then an additional 9 states have either expanded or are planning to expand Medicaid eligibility. During this time, insurance enrollment increased by 16 million, resulting in a 40 percent decline in the uninsured rate from 20.5 percent in 2013 to 12.2 percent in 2016 (Kaiser Family Foundation, 2017). Despite these early gains in enrollment, premiums also steadily rose (ASPE Office of Health Policy, 2017), and 2016 and 2017 were marked by instability as a number of insurers exited the exchanges as a result of unfavorable risk pools created through adverse selection (Wise et al., 2012; Khazan, 2017). Since the enactment of the ACA, its repeal has been a persistent priority for many congressional leaders. Because repeal of the ACA would in principle eliminate the Center for Medicare and Medicaid Innovation (CMMI), repeal proposals called into question the fate of CMMI's VBP demonstrations (Whitman, 2016c).

The MACRA Quality Payment Program

The Medicare Access and CHIP Reauthorization Act (MACRA)—signed into law in 2015—mandated sweeping changes to physician reimbursement under Medicare. The legislation repealed the sustainable growth rate formula and replaced Medicare's various physician quality reporting programs with a single program: the Quality Payment Program (QPP). The stated goals of the QPP are to reform Medicare Part B payments to incentivize higher value care, rather than a higher volume of services. Information presented in this section is current as of August 1, 2018. Given the ongoing revisions to the QPP, some program details will likely change over time.

Eligibility for the QPP

Currently, physicians, physician assistants, nurse practitioners, certified registered nurse anesthetists, and clinical nurse specialists are all eligible to participate in the QPP. Starting in 2019, the Secretary of Health and Human Services has the authority to broaden eligibility to include other types of providers (e.g., physical therapists, nutritionists, clinical social workers). Several categories of eligible providers are exempt from the QPP requirements; these include providers in their first year of billing Medicare and providers meeting the low-volume and low-dollar (i.e., low Medicare billings) threshold exemptions.

In 2017, the low-volume threshold exemption applied to providers with less than $30,000 in annual Medicare charges, or those seeing fewer than 100 Medicare patients, in the prior 12 months. In 2018, the exemption criteria were liberalized to apply to providers with less than $90,000 in annual Medicare charges or those seeing fewer than 200 Medicare patients. However, for individual providers who are part of a group practice, exemption from the QPP is determined by the Medicare billing patterns of the entire group. Therefore, if a group collectively exceeds the low-volume exemption threshold, all individual providers in that group are considered nonexempt from the QPP—even if some of them individually see a small number of Medicare patients.

Under the QPP, eligible and nonexempt providers caring for Medicare beneficiaries can choose to participate in one of two pathways: the Merit-Based Incentive Payment System (MIPS) or Advanced Alternative Payment Models (AAPMs). Each pathway is described in greater detail below. Nonexempt providers who opted out of the QPP in 2017 will receive a negative payment adjustment of 4 percent of their Part B payments in 2019, and the size of the penalty will increase over time.

Merit-Based Incentive Payment System

MIPS functions similarly to a PFP model: The underlying payment model is FFS, and payments are adjusted according to quality and cost measures. Each practice receives a "MIPS Score," a weighted average of their performance in four domains. Three of the four domains are modifications of existing Medicare quality incentive programs: Quality (previously the Physician Quality Reporting System), Cost (previously the Value-Based Payment Modifier), and Advancing Care Information (previously the Medicare EHR Incentive Program). The fourth domain, Improvement Activities, is new. Providers must report on their performance on measures and activities in each of these domains, with the exception of the Cost domain, which is calculated by CMS via claims. Over time, the plan is for the Quality and Improvement Activities weights to decrease, while the Cost weight increases: In other words, cost of care will have an increasing influence on providers' overall performance in MIPS.

A key feature of MIPS is the delay between reporting periods and payment periods. Providers' performance data in a given calendar year is used to adjust their payments two calendar years later; that is, performance data from 2017, the first reporting year[2] in MIPS, will be used to adjust payments in 2019, and so forth. Providers who do not satisfy the minimum MIPS Score performance threshold—which was a score of 3 in 2017 and 15 in 2018—will receive a penalty. Providers who did not meet the minimum threshold in the 2017 reporting year will be penalized by losing up to 4 percent of their Part B payments in 2019; for the 2020 payment year, the penalty increases to up to 5 percent; by the 2022 payment year, it will increase to a maximum of 9 percent. Conversely, providers who exceed the minimum performance threshold are eligible for bonuses: up to 4 percent of Part B payments in payment year 2019, up to 5 percent in payment year 2020, and up to 9 percent in payment year 2022. Providers with

---

[2]   CMS commonly uses the term "performance year" regarding MIPS. Throughout this report, however, we use the terms "reporting year" and "performance year" interchangeably.

exceptionally strong performance are eligible for an additional bonus, up to but not exceeding 10 percent of their Part B payments. Finally, starting in 2026 MIPS participants will receive an annual baseline payment update of 0.25 percent.

Advanced Alternative Payment Models

Each year CMS determines which models qualify as AAPMs. To qualify for an AAPM, practices or physician organizations must meet the following criteria: 50 percent of participants use an EHR; the practice reports quality measures comparable to MIPS and adjusts provider payments based on these measures; and the practice bears some financial risk if cost and quality targets are not met. Currently, an individual provider is considered to be participating in an AAPM if she receives at least 25 percent of her Part B payments, or sees at least 20 percent of her Medicare patients, through an AAPM. These thresholds are slated to increase over time. By 2023, a provider must receive at least 75 percent of her Part B payments from an AAPM to qualify as a participant (Castellucci, 2017b).

As with MIPS, there is a two calendar-year delay between the performance and payment periods. In the 2019 and 2020 payment years, AAPMs that did not meet cost and quality targets in 2017 and 2018, respectively, stand to lose the lesser of either 8 percent of Part A and B revenues, or 3 percent of expected expenditures (though for the medical home models that qualify as AAPMs, such as CPC+, the share of revenue at risk is smaller). AAPM participants that achieve their cost and quality targets will receive a positive payment adjustment of 5 percent in the payment years from 2019 to 2024. Starting in 2026, AAPM participants will receive an annual baseline payment update of 0.75 percent (i.e., higher than for MIPS).

A third, hybrid option under the QPP is MIPS Advanced Payment Models (APMs). MIPS APMs are entities that base payments to their member organizations or physicians on cost and quality measures but do not satisfy all the criteria for AAPMs. These entities are eligible for the same bonuses as MIPS practices, but they benefit from simplified reporting requirements and automatic full credit for Improvement Activities.

Changes to the QPP

Since its inception, the QPP has undergone numerous changes, many of which aim to decrease the reporting burden on participating practices and physicians, especially small or rural practices that might face high administrative costs of compliance in the short-term. Some notable changes to the original MIPS rules include the exemption of a growing number of small practices through an increase in the low-volume threshold (Dickson, Muchmore, and Livingston, 2016); rewarding practices that serve an especially medically complex population or a high number of dual-eligibles by adding additional points to their MIPS scores; and permitting small practices to band together as "virtual groups" and report as a single entity, thereby allowing them to share the administrative burdens of reporting (Panjamapirom and Lazerow, 2017). In addition, the program's emphasis on cost containment has increased. Whereas the 2018 proposed rules originally delayed the use of the cost measures until the 2019 reporting period, the 2018 final rules introduced a 10 percent weight on cost measures, with a plan to increase this weight to 30 percent by the 2019 reporting period (Panjamapirom and Lazerow, 2017). The recently released proposed rules for 2019 include the removal of certain process-based quality measures that, per CMS, "clinicians have said are low-value or low-priority, that have a greater impact on health outcomes" (Federal Register, 2018).

The combined effect of the low-volume exemptions and the exemption from MIPS of providers who participate in AAPMs has meant that only 40 percent of the 1.5 million clinicians who bill Medicare are currently eligible for MIPS (Dickson, 2018c).

Providers' Attitudes Toward the MACRA QPP

A number of published articles have explored providers' attitudes toward the MACRA QPP. A general theme emerging from these articles is that there is much uncertainty and anxiety across practices in terms of how to meet the requirements of the QPP (Muchmore, 2016; *Health Management Technology Magazine*, 2017). Key concerns include the administrative burden associated with a growth in quality reporting requirements (Castellucci, 2017b; Van Dyke, 2017; Kocot et al., 2017), the validity of the quality measures used (MacLean, Kerr, and Qaseem, 2018), the complexity of the QPP rules (Wolinsky, 2016), the increasingly difficult criteria that must be satisfied to qualify as an AAPM participant (Castellucci, 2017b), and the disproportionate burden on solo and small practices that have limited capital to support the fixed costs of compliance (Wax, 2017; Kocot et al., 2017). Prior experience in other programs such as the Physician Quality Reporting System (PQRS) and Meaningful Use might contribute to preparing physicians for QPP (Kocot et al., 2017). Industry analysts have predicted that larger numbers of physicians may move from independent practices to employment models to avoid the administrative burdens of compliance, and they have questioned whether some physicians will choose to retire early or stop caring for Medicare patients rather than comply with the QPP (Wolinsky, 2016).

Some practice leaders, however, have a more positive outlook on the QPP, and they have embraced it as part of a growing trend toward population health management, which they view as inevitable (Van Dyke, 2017). For the first reporting year of MIPS, 91 percent of eligible clinicians submitted quality data (Dickson, 2018a).

In response to physicians' concerns about the burdens of the QPP, CMS has made several significant changes to the program, reactions to which have been mixed. The increase in the low-volume exemption threshold for reporting year 2018—which exempted approximately 123,000 more physicians from MIPS (Panjamapirom and Lazerow, 2017)—was welcomed by providers who were concerned about their readiness for MIPS. In contrast, practices that were more experienced with value-based payment were strongly opposed to these changes, in part due to concerns that the size of the potential bonuses they could earn would be reduced. The QPP is designed to be a budget-neutral program; so if fewer penalties are collected, fewer dollars will be available to pay bonuses. Given that many of the practices exempted by the threshold change would likely have been subject to penalties, the size of the bonus pool has been smaller than anticipated. Under the original proposed rules for the QPP, it was estimated that the size of the bonus pool in 2019, the first payment year, would be $833 million, but this fell to $199 million when the $30,000 low-volume threshold was established; for 2020, the projected bonus pool is even lower, at $118 million (Dickson, 2018c). These developments have frustrated providers who made significant financial investments to comply with MIPS, and they are now concerned that they will not recoup these outlays in bonus payments (Dickson, 2018d).

Physicians are not alone in their concerns about the MACRA QPP. In March 2018, the Medicare Payment Advisory Commission (MedPAC) recommended eliminating the MACRA QPP and replacing it with an alternative approach to value-based care. In making this recommendation, MedPAC cited the following concerns: the ability of practices to select which measures they report (from a set of hundreds of measures) will result in invalid comparisons of practices reporting on different measures; most clinicians do not have sufficient volume in a year for their performance metrics to represent reliable, valid measures of the quality of care they provide; the measures do not reflect the team-based nature of medical care; and the reporting requirements are too burdensome (Crosson et al., 2018).

Methods

To describe the evolution of payment models and their longitudinal effects on physician practices since 2014, this project used the same qualitative multiple case study method as our 2014 study, relying primarily on semistructured interviews (Yin, 2014; Friedberg, Chen, et al., 2015). Whenever possible, we sought to interview the same individuals and organizational representatives that we interviewed in 2014. We then supplemented the sample with new interviewees, aiming to collect data on payment models and practices that emerged since 2014. As before, we included a relatively large total number of cases (31 physician practices in six markets) because we wanted to capture a diversity of practice sizes, specialties, and ownership models—an approach that allowed us to assess whether findings replicated across cases and offered a degree of generalizability (Yin, 2014). To collect updated data on market context, we also interviewed market observers from the same categories we used in 2014: leaders of health plans and hospitals operating in the market, state or county medical societies, and state Medical Group Management Association (MGMA) chapters.

Data Collection

Overview

Between January 2018 and June 2018, we gathered data from 84 interviewees nested within 31 physician practices in six markets throughout the country, each roughly defined by its metropolitan statistical area: Little Rock, Arkansas; Orange County, California; Miami, Florida; Boston, Massachusetts; Lansing, Michigan; and Greenville, South Carolina. We also conducted interviews with 32 market observers between December 2017 and May 2018: eight health plan leaders, 10 hospital and hospital system leaders, 10 state and local medical society leaders, and four MGMA chapter leaders.

We also administered to each physician practice a brief financial questionnaire (instrument available in the online Appendix) that collected data on payer mix and participation in alternative payment models. We used questionnaire responses to help interpret interview data.

Market Selection

We selected the same six geographic markets as in our 2014 study.[1] We originally chose these six markets from the 12 communities included in the Community Tracking Study/Health

---

[1] For more detail, please see the Methods section of our 2014 study: M. W. Friedberg, P. G. Chen, C. White, O. Jung, L. Raaen, S. Hirshman, E. Hoch, C. Stevens, P. B. Ginsburg, L. P. Casalino, M. Tutty, C. Vargo, and L. Lipiski (2015). *Effects of Health Care Payment Models on Physician Practice in the United States.* Santa Monica, Calif.: RAND Corporation.

Tracking Physician Survey (CTS/HTPS) to maximize diversity on local provider market concentration, payer market concentration, hospital roles, and payment models.

Market Context: Sample of Interviewees

Within each market, we invited market observers in each of the following categories to participate in semistructured interviews: leaders of state and county medical societies and Medical Group Management Association chapters (to gather information on the history of the market and the evolution of physician practices); leaders of health plans with significant market share (to gather information on payment models used by each plan and changes—and reasons for changes—to these models); and leaders of hospitals with significant market share (to gather information on payment models in which each hospital participates, changes in these models, and changes in relationships between the hospital and physician practices in the market).

For each type of market observer, we initially invited the same interviewees who participated in our 2014 study. When an organization's leadership had changed since 2014, we sought to interview its new leader. We conducted 24 market observer interviews total; several included multiple interviewees.

Practice Sample

As in 2014, we defined a physician practice as a business entity that accepted payment to support clinical care delivered by physicians. Practices could range from independent solo practices to large corporations (with or without inclusion of hospitals or other facilities). Some independent practices were affiliated with (but not owned by) larger organizations such as independent practice associations (IPAs) and physician hospital organizations (PHOs). We counted all sites of a given business entity (e.g., a large medical group with multiple locations) as a single physician practice.

Our initial practice sample consisted of all 34 practices that participated in our 2014 study. Within these practices, we sought to interview the same individuals as we did in 2014 whenever possible. Because some practices declined to participate in the current study, or could not participate independently because they no longer met our study definition of a physician practice (e.g., they had been acquired by larger practices and therefore ceased to exist as a distinct practice), we supplemented the sample with new physician practices based on nominations from market observers (i.e., a snowball sampling strategy). As before, we did not require physician membership in either the AMA or the corresponding state medical society for potential inclusion. In seeking nominations, we specified our interest in practices with a range of experiences in alternative payment programs and a variety of specialties, sizes, and ownership models.

In total, we invited 71 physician practices to participate in the study (the 34 original practices plus 37 supplemental practices), aiming for 6 practices in each market. At the close of data collection, 31 physician practices agreed to participate. Of these, 18 had participated in our 2014 study. Some practices had multiple sites, and we interviewed physicians in 41 distinct practice sites.

As shown in Table 1, the sample was diverse in terms of practice size, ownership, and specialty. However, we were unable to sample practices with every *combination* of dimensions (as represented by the empty cells), partially because certain combinations are relatively uncommon (e.g., a large single-specialty practice or a small multispecialty practice).

Table 1
Physician Practice Sample

Practice Size	Physician-Owned or Partnership			Hospital or Corporate Owner		
	Multispecialty	Primary Care	Single Subspecialty	Multispecialty	Primary Care	Single Subspecialty
Large (> 50 physicians)	4			6		
Medium (10–49 physicians)		1	5	1	1	2
Small (< 9 physicians)		7	3		1	

NOTE: Single subspecialty practices included Cardiology, Gastroenterology, General Surgery, Neurology, Ophthalmology, Orthopedic Surgery, and Psychiatry.

Data Collection: Semistructured Interviews

To create interview guides for the current study, we began with the interview guides that we used in our 2014 study and added items that specifically queried changes in payment models since 2014. For physician practice interviewees, we also asked for updates on their experiences with the payment models they had described in 2014. The interview guides are available in the online Appendix.

Within each physician practice, we asked to speak with at least one practice leader who had knowledge of practice finances and operations and at least one frontline physician providing clinical care. Of the 84 physician practice interviewees, 25 were practice leaders who were not clinicians, and 59 were physicians (some of whom were practice leaders). Each interview lasted 45 to 60 minutes and was recorded and transcribed with interviewee consent. Nearly all physician practice interviews were conducted in person by study staff who visited the practice sites. We conducted interviews with market observers via telephone.

Data Analysis

An eight-person multidisciplinary team consisting of two general internists, one general pediatrician, and five policy researchers performed the qualitative analyses. Six of the eight members of the data analysis team also performed site visits and conducted the semistructured interviews and were thus familiar with the data.

As in our 2014 study, we developed a code structure using inductive procedures to generate insights based on the views the study participants had expressed (Bradley, Curry, and Devers, 2007). The qualitative analysis team met weekly throughout the project to discuss each site visit in detail, expand and refine a running list of key concepts identified from each interview, and organize and define relationships between identified concepts. The running list of concepts served as the initial codebook for qualitative analysis.

Using this codebook, the team coded the interview transcripts, using the constant comparative method to ensure that themes were consistently classified, while allowing for expansion and refinement of codes (Bradley, Curry, and Devers, 2007). Following the multiple case study framework (Yin, 2014), we coded each interview with a physician practice respondent in the context of the payment models to which the practice was exposed (a practice-level variable).

The qualitative analysis team used essential components of consensual qualitative research to code the interview transcripts, including agreeing on the meaning of the data and auditing the work of each qualitative coder to ensure consistency (Kvale, 1996; Hill et al., 2005). Each member of the coding team coded a set of interview transcripts independently. Two senior members of the coding team cross-checked the work of the other coders. Any coder could suggest new codes, and codebook addition or refinement decisions were made by consensus after discussion by the qualitative analysis team. We used Dedoose Version 4.12 (SocioCultural Research Consultants LLC, Los Angeles) to manage and analyze qualitative data.

Limitations

The limitations of our methods reflect the study design. First, because data collection required voluntary investment of time and effort from practice leaders and physicians, it is possible that practices for which study participation would have been a significant financial hardship (e.g., those struggling the most with new payment models) were underrepresented. Second, interviewees might have felt pressure to give answers that they believed would be more "socially acceptable" than their true beliefs, thus introducing social desirability bias. For example, respondents might have been more likely to attribute shared problems (to which they or their organizations might have contributed, in some way) to other parties. Third, practical considerations including the project time line influenced our sampling plan, and we did not seek to reach theoretical saturation. However, we did not identify new major findings toward the end of the data collection period. Fourth, the market observers who nominated practices for inclusion in the study might have selected practices likely to have a perspective they agreed with. Our inclusion of several types of market observers, including health plan leaders, was intended to mitigate this potential source of bias. Finally, our sample was not nationally representative, so our findings might not generalize to markets beyond those included in the study. A future project, such as a nationally representative survey of physician practices, could estimate the prevalence of the findings reported here.

Update on Study Markets

We gathered contextual information on characteristics of each of the six study markets from leaders of local medical societies, MGMA chapters, health plans, hospitals, and physician practices. These interviewees provided information on market concentration, recent changes to prevailing payment models, and relationships between hospitals and physician practices in the market. The descriptions below are as reported by market observers, without comparison to other data sources. This chapter reviews market context in 2014 (as a baseline) and describes changes from 2014 to 2018 within each market.

Boston, Massachusetts

2014 Market Characteristics
A high percentage of physicians were specialists. Academic hospital-based medical centers and one for-profit hospital chain dominated the service delivery landscape. Outside of teaching hospitals, direct physician employment was rare, but alignment with hospitals was increasing. There were three major commercial health plans—all regional—and Blue Cross Blue Shield of Massachusetts had much greater market share than others. The Alternative Quality Contract (AQC) for HMO enrollees from Blue Cross Blue Shield included shared savings based on global spending, with prominent PFP.

Changes Between 2014 and 2018
Blue Cross Blue Shield of Massachusetts expanded the AQC to its PPO membership; about 60 percent of PPO members and 85 percent of HMO members were included in this payment model. Physician practice affiliation with hospital systems continued to increase, though hospital systems were still largely driven by FFS incentives. Two major independent physician groups remained.

One physician group recently experienced a decrease in its risk-based contracting in favor of FFS. This shift was attributed by group leaders to employers favoring high-deductible PPO products over HMOs, resulting in increased emphasis on volume at the practice level.

The Boston market overall continued to undergo significant changes. During the fieldwork period for this project, Massachusetts Medicaid (MassHealth) implemented a mandatory ACO for its beneficiaries, and a planned merger between two large hospital systems and their affiliated physician groups was undergoing regulatory review.

Greenville, South Carolina

2014 Market Characteristics

A high percentage of physicians were employed by hospitals, and many others were loosely affiliated. There were few independent physicians and no large independent multispecialty groups or IPAs. Given the high rate of physician-hospital alignment, there was substantial interest in establishing ACO agreements. Blue Cross Blue Shield had 60 percent of the commercial market, and PPOs with high rates of patient cost-sharing were common. There were two large and two small hospital systems serving the market.

Changes Between 2014 and 2018

Most physician practices were employed by one of two health systems, while a small and shrinking number of primary care groups remained loosely affiliated or independent. Such practices reported that much of this consolidation was driven by recent payment reforms, including the MACRA QPP. In contrast, major subspecialty groups generally remained independent, largely untouched by alternative payment models.

Lansing, Michigan

2014 Market Characteristics

There were many small practices and few moderate or large groups. There was increasing physician employment by hospitals. Larger practices had achieved or were seeking medical home recognition. Blue Cross Blue Shield had 70 percent of the commercial market, and its HMO subsidiary had an additional 10 percent of the market. Two major hospital systems made up 90 percent of the market; the smaller of these hospital systems focused on profitable specialty lines.

Changes Between 2014 and 2018

Hospital employment of physicians continued to increase. Falling payment rates and lack of access to capital were cited as reasons why physician practices sought employment with hospitals. The same two major hospital systems present in 2014 continued to dominate the market. However, the smaller of the two increased its purchasing of independent physician practices and partnered with the local university hospital, enlarging its market share substantially.

Blue Cross Blue Shield of Michigan continued to dominate the commercial market. Alternative payment model penetration increased. Primary care practices participated in both CPC+ and commercial Blue Cross Blue Shield medical home designation programs. Blue Cross Blue Shield of Michigan also engaged most of its PPO market in the Physician Group Incentive Program (PGIP), an APM in which FFS payment rates were modified based on prior-year performance on cost and quality measures.

Miami, Florida

2014 Market Characteristics

Most physicians were in small independent primary care practices or specialty groups of fewer than 50 physicians who admitted patients to multiple hospitals. The payer market was relatively unconcentrated with no dominant payer. There were large nonprofit and for-profit systems, but none was dominant in the market as a whole. Hospitals were historically geographically segmented with little competition, but there was greater competition to attract wealthy patients.

Changes Between 2014 and 2018

Miami saw growth in large specialty practices, and hospitals bought many smaller practices, leaving fewer solo practitioners. This consolidation was reportedly driven by small practices' lack of access to capital and the expertise necessary to implement EHRs, as well as desire for better bargaining positions in contract negotiations with payers. There was also a robust market for consultants to help with everything from contract negotiations and mergers to EHR implementation and MACRA QPP compliance. There was growth in concierge practices and physicians seeking hospital employment.

Reimbursement in the commercial market was largely through FFS, and commercial payment rates were generally below Medicare rates. Some practices engaged in both Medicare and commercial ACOs (primarily upside-only risk models), and some were successful in receiving performance bonuses.

Orange County, California

2014 Market Characteristics

Many physicians were in solo or small practices that each joined multiple IPAs to contract for HMO patients. However, the number of IPAs each physician practice joined was decreasing. There was no dominant payer. Anthem Blue Cross had 33 percent of the market, and Kaiser 20 percent. There was an unconsolidated hospital sector, with three systems making up 50 percent of the market. There was growing interest in hospital-physician affiliations.

Changes Between 2014 and 2018

There was significant hospital consolidation, as well as increased affiliation with larger physician groups. Some solo and small practices also merged or joined larger groups. Physician groups still joined multiple IPAs, but some changed their affiliations from 2014. While some physicians were employed by hospital foundations, a greater number were affiliated but not employed.

Some commercial HMOs decreased reimbursement to close to Medicare rates. Many PPO plans contracted with increasingly narrow networks due to employer pressure for lower-cost plans. As one market observer put it, "What people want is a PPO product that can be managed like an HMO product," resulting in narrow-network PPOs at HMO-like prices for consumers, but without HMO-like management of patients. Medicaid enrollment increased, with over 20 percent of the market. Less than one-third of the market overall was reimbursed through FFS.

Little Rock, Arkansas

2014 Market Characteristics

Most physicians worked in small, independent practices, with relatively few large multispecialty groups. Blue Cross Blue Shield had nearly 70 percent of the commercial market, and two other plans divided the bulk of the remainder. There were three large hospital systems, all of which were statewide referral centers. The Arkansas Medicaid program had recently initiated bundled payment and medical home programs for multiple specialties.

Changes Between 2014 and 2018

Physician practices were increasingly being acquired by hospitals. Physician employment was increasing toward 50 percent. Larger health systems were consolidating into clinically integrated networks to prepare for participation in ACO models. Two competing large health systems had recently established a joint MSSP Track 1+ (risk-bearing) ACO.

Blue Cross remained the dominant commercial payer in the market, and smaller plans generally followed Blue Cross's lead in payment models. State legislation curtailed the bundled payment initiatives present in 2014. Risk-bearing agreements were largely upside-only. CPC+ medical home program activity had expanded in the state.

Arkansas expanded Medicaid eligibility through a Section 1115 waiver and enrolled the expansion population in commercial plans available on the exchange. These expansion plans reimbursed providers at rates higher than traditional Medicaid but lower than their other commercial products. There was a new mandatory managed care initiative through Medicaid for patients with developmental disabilities or severe and persistent mental illness.

Persistent Findings: Challenges Associated with Alternative Payment Models

Overview of Findings

Our 2014 study identified several key challenges facing physician practices that were participating in alternative payment models. At the practice level, alternative payment models increased the importance of data and data analysis (as well as data deficiencies and inaccuracies). At times, alternative payment models also conflicted with each other and with government regulations, complicating practices' ability to respond in a constructive manner. For individual physicians, core clinical activities were unchanged, but participation in alternative payment models had increased the volume of nonclinical activities, particularly documentation needs. Finally, our 2014 study identified problems with data integrity and timeliness, errors in payment model execution (including inaccurate measure specification and patient attribution), incomprehensible incentives, and concerns about measure validity, all of which limited the effectiveness of alternative payment models.

All the challenges described by respondents in 2014 persisted as challenges in the current study. In particular, issues related to data continued to constrain practices' ability to understand and improve their performance. Operational errors in payment models also continued to be a source of frustration for physician practices, at times with financial consequences. In some cases, these negative experiences reduced practices' future willingness to participate in alternative payment models, even when offered by different payers. Because physician practices typically participated in multiple payment models from a variety of payers, challenges related to interactions between payment models also persisted.

Detailed Findings

Data Issues

Concerns about data ranged from worries about practices' analytic capabilities to the dangers of inaccurate, incomplete, or untimely data. Concerns about inaccurate, incomplete, or untimely data applied not only to the performance data themselves (i.e., claims data from payers) but also to having access to the benchmarks and targets practices were expected to meet.

Interviewees in all markets described how APMs increased the importance of practices' data management and analytic capabilities, both of which are necessary for reporting requirements and patient care improvement efforts. From the physician perspective, this challenge was particularly acute for those in small and/or independent practices.

Several market observers also described the challenges involved in providing support and education related to the data requirements that practices need for participation in alternative payment models. Some expressed concern that many practices did not have the resources to pay for the consultants and data analysts that were required, while others noted that even if practices did find resources to support consultants and data analysts, requirements were continually changing, making these ongoing expenses.

New Data and Analytic Needs

Practices described lacking the data and analytic capacity necessary to optimize their participation in alternative payment models. In many instances, a single dataset simply did not exist to help the practice assess its own performance on measures required in alternative payment models. One respondent described the added challenge of not having resources to pay for access to much-needed data:

> We have a couple of spreadsheets that we transfer data into so that we can see how we're doing. But there is no other database of all the information. . . . I don't think there's a practice out there that's not a part of something like an ACO or an MSO [management services organization] that has a data repository where you can manipulate the data . . . there's another group of people that have data repositories and can manipulate the data for ACOs. You have to pay for that. . . . We don't have the money to do that.
> —administrative leader of a large single-specialty practice
> participating in several ACOs

Practices also noted that as data requirements changed over time, data infrastructure that worked previously could become inadequate under current reporting pressures. A respondent whose practice had long participated in alternative payment models with quality reporting requirements described this challenge:

> Dollars in quality are significantly less than what they used to be . . . it's much harder to get to those targets because . . . everybody's working on it, so it just gets harder. . . . We began to get very frustrated with the 85 different databases we had of the same electronic record, because although the vendor said everybody could talk to each other, it was not a real unified record. . . . What they really wanted was a unified system . . . to be able to communicate through one record, be able to see each other's notes. . . . We're really trying to make it a record that will really help us improve quality. We are not there yet.
> —physician leader (and practicing physician) in a large multispecialty practice
> participating in capitation and ACOs

Incomplete or Inaccurate Data

Accessing even relatively straightforward internal data could be a challenge, as described by a respondent when asked how many patients the practice currently served:

> Well, quite honestly, we don't know that, and I'll tell you why. No chart hygiene was ever done. And what I call chart hygiene is that every year you go in and you look at your medical record and you run a list of who hasn't been here in three years. You go in and shut their record down so the whole system's not counting them . . . you can delimit what you're running. . . . He ran it the other day and he thinks it's somewhere around 36,000. I don't know. I don't trust that number, really.

> —administrative leader of a small primary care practice
> participating in CPC+ and an ACO program

In some cases, the accuracy of the measure goal was in question. For example, one respondent was wary of the accuracy of payer-provided benchmarks because of prior experience in another APM, in which seemingly minor data elements were changed, causing a major shift in the practice's performance. As the practice began ramping up participation in a new payment model (an MSSP), the respondent expressed concern about the transparency of the data feeding into the development of the benchmark:

> I think the problem is the benchmark. We pretty much know on a fairly reasonably lagged basis what the claims data is, but we don't know what the benchmark is against what you were going to be measured so that's the issue . . . because of the elements that go into building the benchmark, you don't always know are they all true and relevant . . . are they truly based on information that's reliable and verifiable, I think is more the issue.
> —administrative leader of a hospital system with owned and affiliated practices
> participating in an ACO, MSSP, and PFP

Data Timeliness

Practices repeatedly emphasized the need for timely data. When data were late, they found it difficult to reconcile the data or utilize the data to make necessary mid-course corrections to improve or optimize their own performance. Two respondents described their experience with delays in data from an ACO program:

> They're so late in getting you data that it's hard to tie them together, so you just have to accept that it's true and real. . . . We are concerned about how verified it is. . . . If you just look at the first three months, you might only be looking at half of the actual payments because of the delays in people sending bills, the delays in them getting adjudicated by Medicare . . . you have to wait until everything gets sort of billed out and that can take you at least six months. . . . That's the biggest downside in these value-based things, is that there is no tie-in between what they're judging this on where we can get really rapid turnover of data. It's just not there yet. And it definitely limits you.
> —physician leader of a hospital system with owned and affiliated practices
> participating in MSSP

> With the MSSP program . . . it's March 2018, and we really don't have our benchmark yet for 2017, so it's hard to really know from a finance perspective how to track how you're performing under those arrangements. So you're doing it a little bit blind . . . the finance people at the hospital particularly would say that they'd like to be able to have a better handle financially on how we're performing under these arrangements rather than having them wait till six months after the year's over and them be surprised. So I think that that's one of the issues that from a hospital perspective we've found with the Medicare programs.
> —administrative leader of a hospital system with owned and affiliated
> practices participating in MSSP

Another respondent voiced a similar concern about data from a commercial payers' PFP program, in which late identification of performance measures, targets, and patients in need of service impaired the practice's ability to meet performance targets and provide care for patients:

We've had three months in this year, [. . . and] they're supposed to give us a list of what we need to do this year for our patients . . . [but] we still don't know what we're supposed to do on these patients. Are we supposed to get mammograms on them? Because they're supposed to give us a list of who needs what, and it was supposed to be done two days ago, and they said, "Oh, it's not going to be done until the next refresh, which is next month." So we're going to go a quarter of the year into the program, without really having the data to actually do what we were supposed to do. So all we can do is guess. . . . It just would be nice at the beginning of the year, at the very beginning, the first of the year, or let's say in December of the previous year, if they just said, "This is what we're measuring. So as you're seeing your patients here, why don't you start working on this?"

—physician owner of a small primary care practice participating in PFP programs

Operational Errors

Some practices described operational errors in the implementation of APMs. Such errors had resulted in nonpayment of earned bonuses, affecting practices' willingness to participate in future APMs. For example, one respondent interviewed both in 2018 and in 2014 described a data error in a Medicaid bundled payment program that resulted in their practice not receiving an earned bonus. As reported in 2014, the practice had identified the error, and the payer agreed one had been committed:

We remapped how we were going to take care of these patients. We wrote a new treatment plan, and we said we were going to get everyone back into the clinic and see them within one week after discharge . . . and then, we went live, [and], for the most part, we've always fallen into the favorable category, that we should get some money back from the [health plan], but we haven't. . . . So, we figured something must be wrong and, oh, it took us forever, but we finally got through to [the health plan], and they said, "Oh, yeah, something is wrong." This was a year ago . . . but I'm still not certain if it's corrected. . . . I'm suspicious that it's not yet. But I'm challenged because it's hard for me to figure out if we've been on the mark all the time or not. It's been very, very difficult running it down.

—subspecialist physician, hospital-affiliated small single-subspecialty practice

In our 2018 interview, this respondent reported that the error had *not* been corrected in 2014, and in fact was never corrected:

[In 2014] the real issue was . . . they had incorrect data. Because to qualify for a bonus, you had to make certain all the patients were on an ACE inhibitor or an angiotensin receptor blocker . . . and they said we were hitting the target like 75 percent of the time, or 50 percent of the time, and then you could also see what the data was for all the other aggregated hospitals and I saw that they were even lower than us . . . so I was suspicious that something was wrong, and then we audited some of our charts. And that's when we reported to, you know, we brought this to the attention of the state. And they said, "Yeah, we'll get on top of it. We'll correct it." But nothing ever happened. And we would keep getting the reports back, and they'd say the target wasn't met. It was never fixed. . . . I gave up, and I think the hospital leadership gave up.

This particular state's Medicaid bundled payment program ended before 2018. Despite the operational error in this APM, the respondent reported that the effort was worthwhile because the quality of patient care had truly improved—even if the practice never received credit for the improvement. However, as the respondent also noted, this negative experience made other practice leaders more reluctant to participate in a subsequent Medicare bundled payment initiative:

> [Regarding Medicare bundled payments,] I was probably one of the most anxious about that and said, "Guys, you know, we got to get together on this and get going." . . . Perhaps because everything fell apart with the state initiative before, I wasn't getting a lot of traction. . . . They put it on hold.

This example details the experience of a single practice, but multiple practices of different sizes, spanning multiple markets, reported similar challenges due to operational errors in other APMs. For example, a practice in a different market described how a seemingly innocuous change in the way that a baseline was calculated caused their practice to suddenly incur a significant penalty in an APM in which they previously had been successful. This unintended penalty occurred despite close contact with the APM sponsor:

> My team spent many hours on the phone with some brilliant people at [the payer], trying to understand what all the factors were that gave us this big hit. . . . Some of it had to do with the fact that they changed the way they did the baseline. . . . They changed the methodology around the counties, and what the benchmark was . . . we just couldn't make it on that. . . . We really got significantly hurt by the change in their benchmark. . . . [It was] totally unintentional, totally baffled [the payer] and didn't make them happy, because they didn't want us to drop out. We were one of their high-performing groups.
> —physician leader (and practicing physician) in a large multispecialty practice participating in a shared savings model

Within our sample, only physicians and leaders of physician practices described such operational errors in APM implementation. Other market observers did not mention them. Some physician practice leaders noted that without carefully tracking their performance and expected payments or penalties (i.e., keeping their own set of books), these operational errors might have gone unnoticed.

Interference between Payment Models

Practices also cited another particular challenge arising from alternative payment models: the potential for interactions or interference between payment models. In some cases, the conflict between payment models was the result of different incentive structures imposed by different payers and the inherent difficulty of moving from a volume-based to a value-based system. In other cases, the conflict was the result of a lack of alignment in measurement between different payment models.

One respondent noted that the practice overall was beginning to reach an inflection point between volume and value, but individuals within the practice had not yet seen this translate into a financial impact, resulting in challenges to fully participating in either model, and posing a potential risk to the entire practice:

> We feel like we have our feet in two canoes which are moving apart, and so the fundamental nature of the practices is that they're still primarily volume-based payment. The amount of money that's at risk, due to quality or cost of care, is still relatively small. So when it comes to a conversation I'm having with my members, their financial reality is that they

can make up for whatever negative impact there might be . . . by just seeing a few more patients. From the organizational side of things, we have a finite amount of working capital . . . the amount of money that's going to be at risk, now that we have the ACO, it's sort of reached a tipping point for us. At maximal losses, this organization would cease to have working capital in five years.

—administrative leader of a medium-sized primary care practice
participating in an ACO

Several practices described situations in which the transition between value-based and volume-based reimbursement models was further compounded by the need to integrate all physicians into value-based payment models, when many of the rewards were directed at primary care and many of the costs were incurred by specialists. As one respondent put it:

The employed health group of a couple hundred physicians for [health system] in primary care are the ACO-attributed primary care physicians for that ACO. My other 600+ physicians that are medical specialists and surgeons . . . and I've got no "what's in it for me" story . . . because they're not in the ACO. [A]nd so I'm charged with going to a medical specialist or surgeon and saying, look, you know that hysterectomy that you were thinking of doing, well, it's going to cost money and it's probably not indicated but you're going to make money doing it . . . [if you don't do it] you're going to lose money but the ACO is going to benefit. . . . The disconnect in the financial incentives for people to do the best right thing at the right time is still awkward for something like that. . . . It's kind of like going out to dinner with a whole bunch of people and just splitting the check. There's always somebody who orders steak and lobster and somebody who orders chicken, you know somebody saves the money and then somebody doesn't because they just didn't care that much. And the financial incentives that we can offer are so modest that they really aren't a lever.

—physician leader of a large multispecialty practice participating in an ACO

Practices also described facing too many measures, with little to no alignment across payment models. The cacophony of measures was vividly described in 2014 by this respondent:

The PQRS [measures] don't line up particularly well with the meaningful-use ones and, you know, all sorts of other [measures]. It's like [having] 50 people shouting their priorities at you, and then trying to prioritize those into some semblance of order. . . . You lose sight of [whether] this is really having true clinical impact or is this just, you know, like winning the video game? And that's what it starts to feel like after a while when you have a list of 50 things that you're chasing.

—leader of a large multispecialty practice

The lack of alignment was apparent as well in 2018. One respondent highlighted the burden of documentation imposed by attempts to meet all the measure requirements. Significantly, even with additional time spent documenting, this respondent was sure that some component of documentation required for their payment models was missing:

We made a spreadsheet of all of the different insurances we're looking at. . . . It was miserable. . . . We had 20 different groups of columns . . . keeping track of different metrics and all the metrics are different. They may all agree that, hey, we're making sure your patients are getting colonoscopies but one was like, well, have you had a kidney function test if you're on a certain medicine. Are you on an aspirin? And those are the big ones. [A]nd there are also small things. Are you reconciling your medicines every time you're coming in? Well, yes, we ask them. That's one of my nurse's jobs . . . you have to click a certain button in your EMR to say you did it . . . a lot of these things are pretty tedious. [A]nd when you look at me getting through a medical record which I'm going to be quicker than pretty much everybody here at the practice . . . by the time you're done with it . . . there's all this other checkbox stuff that you've got to do . . . I would say just for requirements there it's 30 minutes to an hour out of my day just on documentation and that's with the help from the staff . . . even then we're probably not documenting everything we need to, to meet all those contracts or value-based deals.

—practicing physician in a small primary care practice
participating in an ACO program, PFP programs, and CPC+

A leader of a large multispecialty practice, reflecting on years of tracking performance measures, described the underlying causes of their proliferation and the practice's attempts to harmonize them:

Administrative simplicity means two completely different things whether you're looking at it from the payer's side or from the provider's side. And they're almost antithetical. So administrative simplification to us complicates matters for the payer, and administrative simplification for the payer . . . complicates things for us. . . . The quality side of value-based payment is really a disaster, I would say, and actually MIPS is going to make it worse. [A]nd so, the big thing that we did, which we actually had done by 2014, is we just decided to accept that fact and that we were never going to be able to change it, that everybody was going to make up their own quality measures and they wouldn't be the same across payers . . . and we tried and are still trying to get the commercial payers to kind of go more towards the Medicare model of using clinical data that's derived from actual clinical records. But so far, we haven't been successful.

—physician leader of a large multispecialty practice
participating in ACOs, capitation, and PFP

Uneven Payer Readiness for New Payment Models

In some markets, practices described difficulties they faced in negotiating contracts with payers that were based on anything other than FFS. One practice collected a wide variety of internal quality measurement data, as well as data required for participation in a range of alternative payment models. A respondent from this practice described the frustration of trying to negotiate a contract with a payer that offered only an FFS reimbursement model and had no interest in engaging in the risk contracts suggested by the practice:

The frustrations since 2014 have been with the private insurance trying to say . . . "What percentage of Medicare do you want to get for [zip code]?" . . . It's so antiquated and it's stupid. . . . We show them all this metric data. They don't care. . . . We would love to get into a risk contract relationship. . . . I would love to be a medical home for Alzheimer's, stroke, or TIA [transient ischemic attack] with prevention of stroke, migraine, epilepsy. Because I am a de facto primary care on that individual. That individual won't do anything without clearing it with me first. . . . I'd love to have that, [but] no insurance will recognize it.

—physician leader (and practicing physician) in a large single-subspecialty practice
participating in MIPS

A similar challenge was also reported by local or regional payers hoping to engage federal payers:

> What we hope is that . . . there would be the ability for us to actually engage Medicare into some of the things that we're already doing here. That's been very difficult in the past . . . we've got fairly long-established, pretty effective programs in place, and it would make more sense for Medicare to align with us. It's just been very difficult to do that.
> —commercial health plan leader participating in bundled payments

Some low-cost provider practices noted that participating in alternative payment models was particularly challenging because they had already cut their costs beyond where most payers might have expected. As a result, APMs could not always accommodate them:

> Our health care system . . . it's a low-cost provider. The average ACO person out there is running around $13,000 to $14,000 per year. We were at $9,000, which means we're saving the government several thousand dollars per person per year. We have 25,000 of those people . . . we are a very inexpensive shop to be in. So the world of ACO is you only make money when you cut cost and beat the national trend. But when you're a low-cost provider, it doesn't help much . . . you only win when you take more money out of yourself . . . the model is exhausting . . . when I sit in meetings and I say, "Who would ever agree to take a 2 percent haircut and then beat yourself to . . . if you beat yourself bad enough, have a chance to get half of what you beat yourself with, if you're 100 percent perfect [on quality]?"
> —administrative leader of a large multispecialty practice
> participating in MSSP, capitation, and PFP

Persistent Findings: Physician Practice Strategies Regarding Alternative Payment Models

Overview of Findings

As in 2014, practice leaders and other stakeholders across the study markets implemented a variety of strategies in response to APMs. These included new capabilities and models of care, investments in data and analytics, and internal financial and nonfinancial incentives for individual physicians. Some of these strategies were a continuation of previous efforts (e.g., expanding the roles of care management and care coordination staff), while others involved adding new capabilities (e.g., expanding a primary care practice's scope of care), often enabled by new information technology. Practices also augmented their capabilities to collect and manage data from internal and external sources by investing in staff and information technology.

Despite engagement with new APMs, most practices reported that internal financial incentives for individual physicians had not substantially changed since 2014. Modest bonuses for quality performance remained common, and, with the exception of small, independent practices, individual physician financial incentives based on costs of care were almost non-existent. As in 2014, practice leaders deployed a range of nonfinancial strategies to influence physician decisionmaking, such as internal performance reports intended to appeal to physicians' competitiveness and self-esteem.

Detailed Findings

New Capabilities and Models of Care

Practice leaders in multiple specialties and markets described continuing the investment that had been made in 2014 in response to APMs. For example, one practice invested in capabilities that affected patient care (such as population health), as well as in data capture capabilities (to record hierarchical condition categories [HCCs]):

> We're building an infrastructure. . . . Everything that we explained that's part of the population health and that's part of building the infrastructure. Certified coders, okay, in the HCC, also social workers or people within that education to call the patients, the ARNPs or the physician extenders to actually assist the doctors in the annual wellness visits. That also generates additional revenue. So basically, everything we're doing is building that infrastructure. So, I could tell you that three years ago, we were not there yet. Now, we feel that we're closer and we have a better grip of what we're doing and how to better do risk.
> —administrative leader of a large multispecialty practice

Practice investments in new capabilities also reflected general enthusiasm for certain payment models, especially when respondents believed that a payment model could lead to improvements in patient care:

> This is an opportunity to fundamentally transform care in a way that benefits everyone, our patients first among them. . . . We're clearly responding to external incentives, but I think that when done well—and I'm passionate about that—you can really also improve the quality of care genuinely for these patients and improve the provider experience as well.
>
> —practicing physician in large multispecialty practice

Population Health and Chronic Disease Management

Practice leaders described continuing efforts to more fully implement population health and chronic disease management capabilities associated with PCMH models. These efforts included more extensive staffing and systematic processes for care management and coordination functions for high-risk, complex patients, as well as an emphasis on closing "care gaps" for preventive services for broader populations of patients.

One practice leader noted that participation in alternative payment models for Medicare, Medicaid, and other high-risk populations required a distinct set of capabilities:

> One of the things we've learned is that the management of Medicare populations and commercial populations are quite different. The profile of high-cost patients is quite different . . . and undoubtedly, we'll need a different approach for the Medicaid population. What we've learned from our plan is that there is a one percent frequent-flyer population with multiple comorbidities and very high ED usage and often homeless, and with behavioral health diagnosis, et cetera.
>
> —administrator leader of a hospital system

A number of respondents described an increasing emphasis, since 2014, on the integration of behavioral health in primary care and expanded roles for social workers and related staff to address social determinants of health and health care utilization. Awareness of the opioid epidemic has increased since 2014, and some primary care practices included dedicated substance abuse services among their behavioral health investments.

> So we have a medical home care coordinator program at the clinics, those are expanding, but also their job roles are expanding to include things like social determinants of health assessment and dealing with issues like transportation and referral to agencies. We're embedding behavioral health providers in the primary care clinics, so we have an entire training program online and in person for both therapy folks, as well as the pediatricians, to prescribe medications. We even have a substance abuse program, where we're prescribing medications for opioid withdrawal in some of our primary care practices, that's like world changing.
>
> —physician leader of a large multispecialty practice

Two other capabilities that were the focus of extensive and systematized programs included "closing gaps" in preventive care and transitional care programs, in particular to avoid hospital readmissions. For example, one practice leader described a system for closing gaps in care that involved a team of seven full-time population health coordinators, enabled by an agile electronic registry system:

> We have [. . . a] registry that any physician, any practice, and in looking at the health system as a whole, you can run your list of patients who have care gaps. It's highly filterable, sortable . . . you can pull up all 12,500 diabetics we take care of, and you can order [hemoglobin] A1c's on all of them at the same time. . . . [T]hen we built a team . . . seven full-time population health coordinators. They spend half their time here working together and half their time at the practices, and their job is to bring this registry to life. So they work the registry, find patients with care gaps.
> —physician leader (and practicing physician) in a large practice affiliated with a hospital system

Similarly, a physician discussed his practice's use of an "ACO app" as part of their transitional care program:

> When my patient goes to the emergency room, I receive an alert via the ACO's app. It's going to tell me Mr. Smith is in the emergency room at Hospital [X]. Mr. Smith has been discharged from Hospital [X]. So once I get that, I can talk to the patient or the family and say I am aware that they are there, that I can help. I can provide the doctors with more information. And once I know that the patient was discharged, then me or my staff can call the patient and say, "You've been discharged from Hospital [X]. I'd like you to come Thursday so we can review your medications."
> —physician in a primary care practice participating in a local ACO

One practice organization described changes related to expanding the scope of practice of primary care clinicians (e.g., in dermatology, behavioral health) to avoid unnecessary referrals and to improve both continuity and cost of care:

> We have this concept that we call advanced primary care, so we want to take care that's typically been sent to specialists and try to move it back into the primary care setting, using things like special trainings for pediatricians. So one thing was we wanted to decrease the percent of our patients who had to be referred to outside of the office for dermatology care.
> —physician leader (and practicing physician) in a large multispecialty practice

Staffing and Hiring Strategies

Expanding capabilities often involves substantial hiring, as well as retraining, of staff for new roles. One administrator from a large practice reported receiving $1.4 million in APM bonus money and having "spent all of it . . . on people, and it's made a huge difference." In addition to hiring additional staff in various new roles, several respondents observed a long-term strategy of developing these new groups of staff into fully "fleshed out" and "operational" teams:

> We really have finalized team-based care and family medicine. . . . We fleshed out the team. So we added pharmacists to it, we added some more social workers to it, we put . . . the psychiatrist is in this clinic, we already had a nutritionist. But they've really transitioned from being a pseudo team to really being team based care.
> —administrative leader in a large primary care practice

Some practices experimented with the mix of staff and qualifications for the expanded care management and coordination roles on care teams:

> We've played around a little bit with staff clinical qualifications, so some of them are nurses, some of them are social workers, some of them are neither, it depends on how they adapt to the role, we haven't really found the perfect model. Cost-wise, a nurse is going to be way more expensive than a social worker or an untrained clinical person. So . . . you try to think of how to broadly approach a population where there's not a ton of money in the pot.
>
> —physician leader in a large multispecialty practice

EHR Capabilities

Adapting EHRs to changing APMs was described as an ongoing process. As physician practices have merged into larger networks or been acquired by health systems, a key strategy noted by several respondents was to attempt to move practices to a single EHR platform.

> One of the first things that we did—because when the group came together everybody was either paper charts or different EMRs—we brought all those EMRs into one.
>
> —administrative leader of a large primary care practice

> We began to get very frustrated with the 85 different databases we had, of the same electronic record, because although the vendor said everybody could talk to each other, it was not a real unified record. We went through a very extensive evaluation and what everybody realized . . . they wanted was a unified system, where a primary care doctor could see exactly what was happening in the hospital.
>
> —physician leader (and practicing physician) in a large multispecialty practice

Major new investments in information technology included patient virtual visits (as one administrator of a large practice put it: "We built tech around the virtual visits—they all now have video capabilities with their patients") and a heavy emphasis on dashboards and reporting for internal performance improvement and external payer requirements, including the QPP.

Investments in Data and Analytics

Practices described making a variety of investments in their data management and analytic capabilities in order to perform successfully in APMs.

Data Management

Practices noted that participating fully and successfully in APMs, particularly those involving financial risk, required enhanced data inflows and the ability to manage them:

> In order to do value-based [payment], you've got to have data. . . . If you have no data, you don't go at risk. . . . We've been working with the health plans to let us build an infrastructure. . . . We decided we're going to put money into it and we have a database now that two of our health plans download the claims, real claims. The company that we pay takes everything and puts it together and we know everything about the patient. Everything. Where they went to the ER, how much was it, we know the PMPM [per member per month] by the specialist. . . . The over-users, they just come out . . . we just got to look at the data . . . if you're a cardiologist and I send you a patient, how many times do you see the patient and how many tests do you order? . . . [A]nd we've done that, because of this system,

because data speaks . . . that's where the systems have helped us. IT has got to be the baseline to go at risk . . . because without it, if you go at risk, you're going to lose everything.

—administrative leader of a large single specialty practice
participating in capitation, PFP, and shared savings programs

Data Analytic Capabilities

Finally, practices described improving their analytic capabilities both as a result of and in order
to fully participate in alternative payment models. One respondent described the analytic capabilities needed to participate in capitation and PFP programs:

We follow our own measures . . . I have the target goals right here . . . it's in the system.
We have a scorecard that we're able to look at, and it's updated on a weekly basis. So I can
see where we fall. I can see what measures we're doing really well on, I can see what measures we're still struggling with, and I can dive down to the provider and I can see which
provider is struggling with which measure. I can also identify the missed opportunities that
the provider had. So, you know, of these patients that walked in to see you in the month of
March, or in the month of February . . . hypothetically speaking, 200 were in need of these
screenings and only 100 got screened. So what happened to the other 100? . . . I'm able to
get that report to that level.

—clinic administrator within a large multispecialty practice
participating in capitation and PFP

For some APMs, analytic support came directly from payers, as described by a health plan
leader:

There's a lot of sharing of data as well as analytic reports and performance information. . . .
We have a multidisciplinary team that goes from [payer] to work on site with the clinical
leadership of each organization on a regular basis. . . . As you could imagine, the kind of
data that groups need now is different from what they needed on Day 1 of their [value-
based payment contract]. . . . We still share a full claims data set with complete transparency into what payments are made to different providers in our network so that a provider
who has risk can be a smart shopper when they're referring patients to other parts of the
network and obviously so they can have a 360 view of their patient's care. So we still share
that. But some of our analytic reporting has really evolved from what it was in the early
days.

—health plan leader running PFP and shared savings programs

Physician Incentives and Nonfinancial Interventions

As in 2014, nearly all practices (except very small independent practices) substantially modified the financial incentives they received from payers, rather than passing them directly
through to individual physicians. Some practice leaders still reported that their practices had
only taken "baby steps" toward aligning physician compensation with APMs that involved
substantial financial risk.

Within our sample, FFS was still the dominant internal financial incentive for both
primary care and subspecialist physicians, even in practices with substantial external risk in
shared savings contracts and other APMs. When individual physicians did receive non-FFS
incentives, they were of modest size, framed as upside-only, and typically linked to performance on quality measures. Cost-based individual incentives were almost nonexistent

outside the smallest practices, in which practice and owner or partner physician incomes were inseparable.

Also, as in 2014, practice leaders applied internal nonfinancial tools to individual physicians (e.g., performance feedback and EHR order templates) as strategies for aligning physician decisionmaking with APM-based cost and quality goals.

Financial Incentives for Individual Physicians

Individual physician incentives tended to be framed as upside-only; in some cases, they were tightly linked to underlying FFS-based compensation structures. One respondent described how quality-based incentives were paid on a per relative value unit (RVU) basis:

> I've changed our comp plan for providers . . . we now have 10 percent of the structure at risk. So $2 per RVU are based on HEDIS metrics, $2 per RVU are based on CG CAHPS, and that was decided at a physician level through a physician compensation committee. . . . I'd see that climbing . . . frankly, I'd love to get it to at least 25 percent risk. . . . Right now, our main goal is getting people used to being at risk, when really the structure in Michigan historically is they just get this check from an insurance company saying, "Hey, congratulations! You have $10,000 for your quality scores." So docs view this as a bonus, not really a risk, and you can understand why.
>
> —physician leader of a large multispecialty practice participating in shared savings and PCMH programs

As in 2014, a lack of alternatives to RVUs was cited as an explanation for the persistence of internal FFS, despite practice participation in APMs:

> In general, when you're an environment that's mixed where half your work is fee-for-service and half of it is risk, you still need to have some sort of productivity measure for docs. They're used to [RVUs] and it doesn't make any sense to abandon it.
>
> —physician leader of a large multispecialty practice

Some practices simply divided bonuses equally among physicians, effectively creating group-level performance incentives:

> We're on track with the Medicare ACO to be part of the share tables on that, and so whenever that comes in, that will be distributed at a practice level. Currently we're going to spread that equally over the physicians. That may change, it may not, because we're all pretty much in agreement to make sure that we're all doing the quality metrics and we run our own reports and make sure everybody's doing well with that.
>
> —practicing physician in a small primary care practice

Other practices, especially large multispecialty practices, relied on a wide range of internal financial incentives, even when the entire practice was under the same set of external incentives:

> Well, even with RVUs-based measures it varies enormously across specialties. So primary care we have basically risk-adjusted panel size is a major determinant of compensation. [A]nd for OB or ED or anesthesia, it's about taking shifts and how many shifts you do and what the sort of compensation increment has to be for taking a shift on a night or a weekend or a holiday . . . and you have to have very custom compensation models to kind of live

within the culture and the way in which the practice group is constituted. And . . . we do have a quality incentive program where there's some incremental compensation associated with attainment of quality goals that sort of is layered on top of the routine. . . . But they all vary enormously.

—physician leader of a large multispecialty practice

However, while larger systems and practices tended to shield physicians from the incentives transmitted though external APMs, physicians in smaller independent practices were more exposed to risk-based payment incentives.

The docs in private practice are actually more—they live a net distributable income model—and so they're more directly exposed to the external environment and the external incentives than the employed doctors are.

—physician leader of a large multispecialty practice

Nonfinancial Interventions

As in 2014, practice leaders were wary of passing APM-based financial incentives straight through to individual frontline physicians. As one respondent suggested, practices would sooner try several nonfinancial strategies than pass downside risk to their physicians:

But my big challenge in thinking about how we should be compensating employee doctors is that I don't really know that financial incentives are all that necessary or constructive in terms of changing behaviors. The one thing I know is that if you have financial disincentives—so you have a structure set up where doing the right thing actually causes financial harm—then it's not going to work. You have to try to get those things out of the way.

—physician leader of a large multispecialty practice

Internal strategies such as performance feedback—which could be delivered privately or publicly in the practice—were common among our sample. A practice leader explained how physicians' pride and competitiveness could be used to drive performance improvement:

There's no differential payment of individual member practices, according to their [total medical expenditure] or quality performance, but every one of us got As in college, at least, and a lot of us got As in medical school, and if you send me a report that says that I'm a bottom feeder, I'm pretty bent out of shape, and I want to get those As.

—physician leader and practicing physician in a primary care
practice within large organization

Strategies that involved educating physicians on APMs were described as being less successful:

We've been very aggressive about informing the physicians [about MIPS]. We've had webinars, talks, you know, brought it up at every chance we get because you know to me, tragically, a lot of the physicians went through 2017 seemingly almost unaware that this was a baseline year for their reimbursement in 2019. And I mean we've been lighting ourselves on fire screaming and yelling about it. But it was kind of like the wind wasn't blowing very hard that day and they just didn't really feel like it was that important.

—physician leader in a large multispecialty practice

New Findings: Accelerating Pace of Change in Payment Models

Overview of Findings

Across study markets, multiple practice leaders and market-context interviewees perceived an accelerating pace of change in payment models since 2014. This acceleration, partially driven by implementation of the QPP, capped an already fast-paced decade of successive payment and regulatory changes including PQRS, HITECH, ACA exchange plans, PCMHs, ACOs, and other PFP, shared savings, and episode-based payment programs. This pace of change was challenging for most practices and especially so for small and independent practices. Larger organizations described partially shielding their physicians from payment changes by focusing on long-standing internal goals and by modifying their internal incentives more slowly than the external incentives received from payers.

Market observers noted that even practice management consultants were sometimes unable to keep up with the pace of change, making it harder for small primary care practices in certain markets to find trustworthy advice. Some practice leaders called for a "time out" from further payment changes so that they could better understand how to respond to their current financial incentives.

Sudden or unexpected discontinuations of APMs were particularly challenging for physician practices and other market participants. Respondents attributed these APM reversals to transitions in state and federal political leadership rather than the performance of the models themselves. In some cases, these reversals undermined practices' ability to receive a return on their investments in performance improvement.

In two markets, some practices also reported an unexpected overall shift away from APMs—and back to FFS—in their commercial contracts, perhaps as a consequence of employers increasing their high-deductible health plan PPO offerings. For practices that had developed internal cultures and incentives attuned to APMs, the shift back to FFS undermined physician morale in some cases.

Detailed Findings

Greater Overall Pace of Change

Market observers, physician practice leaders, and frontline physicians described the pace of change in APMs as being faster than anything they had encountered in prior periods of upheaval. Even respondents with decades of industry experience made this observation. For example, one market observer likened the expansion of HMOs in the late 1980s and the implementation of

HIPAA in the 1990s to "big" pills to swallow—yet compared them favorably to the current pace of change:

> [HMOs and HIPAA each] were just kind of like one big pill we had to swallow. Whereas, with the ACA now . . . and PQRS going from an incentive to becoming punitive . . . and Meaningful Use and ICD-10 and now with MIPS this year we have clinical practice improvement activities and then next year we have the resource use piece of MIPS coming in. [A]nd the rules for leaving MIPS to join the APM—or now they're calling them AAPMs— the rules are changing multiple times during the year and all of the different measures that they're following and they care about and the requirements for submitting them. . . . What we're seeing right now is just a lot of these what I would call like big pills to swallow all in a very short time period of the seven to eight years, where it seems like almost every year there's a major shift that you have to make.
>
> —local medical society leader

Challenges Stemming from the Pace of Change

More than one practice leader underscored the challenge of investing staff time to understand— and devise strategies to respond to—new and unfamiliar payment programs. Constraints on staff time were especially acute in smaller practices:

> We're so constrained on staff that the time to investigate [each new payment program], the time to do the thinking, the time to ask questions is hard to come by. And so because of that, I don't think we're doing it as efficiently as we could . . . and we're really just scraping by. And so, A) we're not getting everything done that we could get done, and B) we don't have the time to really think about how to do it better.
>
> —administrative leader of a medium-sized primary care practice

> A lot of the people are trying to align with these new forms of payment, but they don't really know what these new forms of payment are. . . . My staff is four [assistants] and myself. . . . We had to hire a consultant just to get us through this mess because, in spite of what we do, despite all the courses that we take, despite all the webinars that we try to attend, sometimes we have no idea what [payers] want. I mean, seriously, no idea. It's for- eign to us. You try to read one of the papers that the government sends you . . . and at the end of the paper, I don't know what they're talking about. And I am a professional. I'm at least average intelligence and I can't figure out what they're saying.
>
> —physician owner of small single-specialty practice

Some respondents said that vendors and practice management consultants in their mar- kets were having a tough time keeping up with changing payment models, making it harder for practices to get good assistance and advice. One market observer noted that some vendors had retreated to market segments with relatively stable payment models:

> With a lot of the so-called experts that are out there, there's a lot of mismanagement of information. The solo docs especially, I mean, they can't even afford to have their own front-office people go out to get educated at places like the MGMA. . . . I was on the phone earlier today with the owner of a billing company in my area and she was telling me, "I never got involved in any of this stuff because I'm about five years away from retirement, so why would I get involved with all this new ACA, the PQRS, the Meaningful Use, MACRA, and all this stuff? It's just not worth it. It's so complex, it's so complicated. And I

know how to do what I know how to do, so I'm gonna stick with the specialties that don't really depend on that."

—MGMA chapter leader

In some cases, asymmetric change between payment programs and related regulations caught market participants by surprise. For example, several larger practices and hospitals warned that new payment models (e.g., shared savings) encouraged closer physician-hospital relationships that could potentially conflict with anti-kickback regulations:

> Just as these payment models evolve and change, . . . the thing that doesn't seem to change are things like Stark laws. Suddenly having an unintended consequence that now another part of the federal government is saying that you are in violation . . . maybe one paragraph in a ten-page contract suddenly exposes you to, as an organization, to some type of kickback or referral based problem. . . . That's one of the things we struggle with here, in terms of having dialogues with our physicians and adjusting and adapting to new payment models. We think we might know the right thing to do, but then we find out, an attorney tells us that this [new] physician contract now is a problem.

—hospital leader

Practices' Responses to the Pace of Change

In general, interviewees reported that larger practices were better able to respond to changing payment models than were smaller practices. One market observer tied this advantage to the relative size of a practice's internal educational resources: "The larger systems are doing an amazing job reaching out to their physician practices and working with them to be prepared," while in the same market, this respondent noted, turnout for small-practice educational events on payment model changes was alarmingly light:

> We've run a number of programs for individual practicing physicians and I can't tell if the light turnout is a function of people still having their heads in the sand and not recognizing it, or if it's just if they already have been educated [about the MACRA QPP].

—MGMA chapter leader

Another advantage of larger systems was their ability to shield physicians from recent changes in payment models, either by not passing financial incentives straight through to them (as described earlier) or by alleviating the burden of measurement-related data collection:

> One of my biggest roles is to mitigate burnout. Our doctors, in general, are very proud of the quality of care they give, but they don't like to be measured on it. They think "I'm already doing the work, so why do I have to click this box?" . . . But at the end of the day, all these risk contracts require some kind of internal metric of quality. We try to soften that by trying to support practices as much as we can. I think the population health coordinators do probably most of the heavy lifting, when it comes to entering the data in [our EHR] and trying to support the practices.

—physician leader (and practicing physician) in a
large multispecialty practice

Other interviewees—especially those in smaller practices who were unable to insulate their physicians—expressed a desire for a pause, a period of stability to allow new payment models to settle in before making new changes. One solo practitioner asked for a "time out" from additional payment changes:

> We need to call a time out. We need to create a moratorium. . . . Nothing against academics, nothing against new ideas, but before you implement new ideas, let the old ideas get into effect. Many of my colleagues, including me, really have to keep up to understand what is HEDIS, what is MACRA, what is Meaningful Use, when is Meaningful Use phased out, when is MACRA phased in? We don't even have time to take a deep breath in order to digest what is important.
>
> —physician owner of primary care solo practice

Reversals of Alternative Payment Models Challenged Practices

Interviewees in multiple markets reported that, since 2014, certain APMs had suddenly or unexpectedly been discontinued for reasons unrelated to the performance of the models themselves. Transitions in state and federal political leadership were often cited as the cause of these changes. APM reversals were especially challenging for practices that had made investments based on payment models that were suddenly discontinued. For example, bundled payments for acute respiratory infections in one market faded away after a political change, to the surprise and frustration of this practice leader:

> Oh, this is just kind of crazy. Let me think back on it. We were in the bundled payment system for Medicaid [in 2014], and that was proposed by the surgeon general at the time, who was under [the previous] governorship. And the [new] governor came in, he fired the surgeon general. So we have a new surgeon general . . . and so some of those episodes of care have kind of dwindled. . . . [However], it improved care anyway because we strictly forbade the residents to give antibiotics for upper respiratory infections. So I think [bundled payment] made a big difference. . . . [But] it's hard in this day and time to keep anything going and, as you know, with like TV, the focus is about 30 seconds and then you're off to something else.
>
> —physician owner of a small primary care practice

Similarly, the sudden discontinuation of the mandatory Medicare cardiac bundled payment demonstration interrupted the formation of physician-hospital business relationships, sometimes with lingering aftereffects. A market context respondent described planned acquisition of physician practices by hospital systems being halted:

> [Under mandatory cardiac bundled payments, hospitals] were really after the cardiologists . . . and some people have sold and so people were promised to buy or promised they'd be bought and that kind of went on hold and halted. Of course, a lot of people have bad blood because of that. [Cardiologists said], "You promised me to do this and now you're not going to do it," and the hospital said, "Well, I wanted to do it but now I can't do it because it's changed." Same for the orthopedic surgeons.
>
> —medical society leader

To some market observers, these politically-driven reversals in government payment models heightened the importance of engaging private health plans in new payment models, as a means of stabilizing them:

One of the things that I've found over time is, you know, allowing the public programs to lead the market in some of these things is kind of a dangerous proposition, simply because you have administrations that turn over. . . . So if you don't have the private payers out there, at least representing some form of consistency throughout a change in political administration, then you end up taking two steps back sometimes.

—health plan leader

There were also notable shifts back to FFS in two markets, possibly due to employers increasingly offering high-deductible PPOs instead of managed care plans. For physicians who had become accustomed to capitation and shared savings, the rapid transition back to FFS could be unwelcome. A return to volume-based incentives decreased morale enough for this physician to leave a large multispecialty practice:

[Our practice has become] almost exclusively and primarily concerned with volume because of this change [to FFS], which is nothing like we ever were before. And what I am seeing with that change is a decrease in quality, a decrease in patient satisfaction, a decrease in all things that I hold most important, and that's part of why I'm leaving.

—practicing primary care physician within a large multispecialty practice

Practices' Strategies for Handling Future APM Reversals

A minority of practices in our study responded to the possibility of future APM reversals by actively choosing to ignore aspects of payment models that did not align with their preexisting improvement activities or long-term goals. Larger practices with well-developed internal performance improvement and risk management programs were the only ones to report having such strategies. In an illustrative case, one practice leader, when asked about the practice's strategy for MACRA, responded that specific payment program incentives were less important than generally improving quality and managing risk:

How we're basically viewing MACRA right now is we are going to go ahead with some of these [improvement activities], regardless of what MACRA is. I mean, they've changed the rules enough times that frankly with the political climate in Washington at this point . . . we have no idea what we're going to run into, so we're really just trying to do what we think is the right thing for our patients and position ourselves in the future to be able to manage risk, no matter what forms it comes.

—physician leader of large multispecialty practice

New Findings: Increasing Complexity of Payment Models

Overview of Findings

Interviewees from a wide range of practices, markets, and roles said that alternative payment models had become increasingly complex since 2014, citing an expanding range of performance measures, uncertainty about performance thresholds for penalties and rewards, and interactions between different payment models as sources of this complexity. MACRA was a key contributor to this complexity because it introduced new decision points for practices (e.g., the choice between MIPS or an AAPM, or the choice of performance measures from a large menu). Practices of all sizes and specialties said that understanding complex new payment models often entailed a significant investment, either to hire consultants or to build internal capabilities to analyze APMs. In our sample, larger practices and those affiliated with large health systems were able to make these investments, while leaders of smaller, independent practices were more likely to express confusion and disengagement.

For practices that did invest in understanding APMs, the increased complexity of payment models presented new opportunities for financial success. Some of these practices found ways to get more credit for their preexisting quality—without materially changing patient care—by enhancing their documentation and data abstraction practices, thoroughly coding risk adjustment diagnoses, actively managing patient attribution, or purposefully selecting their performance measures to maximize the likelihood of rewards.

Detailed Findings

Challenge: Practices Had Difficulty Understanding Increasingly Complex Payment Models

Many interviewees acknowledged that the increased complexity of payment models made it difficult to understand them. While some physician practices disengaged from new payment models (e.g., ignored MACRA), interviewees more commonly reported the difficulty of trying to understand APMs. One market observer described how challenging this could be for smaller practices:

> I think with the MACRA you have just this very complex point system that very few people are able to kind of really figure out how to properly target and tackle. With clinicians, I mean, clinicians are not mathematicians. They're not business people, generally speaking. You have a high percentage of doctors become business owners, but a very small percentage of them were ever trained in it. So for them to be able to handle these very high-admin type of roles in a practice where if you're just picturing a typical practice—and most practices

are small—you just can't expect them to have people on hand unless they're lucky, unless the doctor's husband happens to be a CPA [certified public accountant] or something like that and can actually dedicate a lot of work to their practice, it's rare that they're going to be able to have the amount of resources internally to handle this stuff.

—MGMA chapter leader

Even some leaders of large health systems reported confusion:

When it comes to the MACRA and the MIPS and all those pieces, I will be the first to tell you I'm somewhat confused as to which set of rules we're playing under. . . . I wish I could speak more intelligently on that, but honestly, I think I've just gotten myself confused.

—leader of a large health system

Strategy: Practices' Investments in Understanding Complex Payment Models

Practices in multiple markets—especially larger ones—reported making substantial investments in their own ability to understand and comply with the requirements of new payment models. Again, this was often particularly challenging for smaller and independent physician practices, as one practice leader explained, in reference to CPC+:

Finding qualified people to run this program has been awful and especially with what the physicians would want to pay to get that quality. You've got to know IT. You've got to know some medicine. You've got to know how to put documents together. You've got to know how to work Excel. You've got to know how to do presentations. You've got to know how to do all of it, you know, the blah-blah—I mean it goes on and on and on—if you're going to do it right. You have to do budgets for CPC. You have to show them how you spent the money. You've got to make sure you're legal doing this or they can come in and take all of your money back from you that you've already used to pay people.

—office manager of medium-sized primary care practice

Practices with greater internal resources, and a willingness to invest them, reported that they could achieve a detailed understanding of complex new payment models. One practice went as far as reverse-engineering a complex payment model by comparing the practice's performance and risk adjustment data to the performance scores that determined its bonuses and penalties:

Interviewee: [We had to figure out] how much of the services that we provide are appropriate because of the risk adjustment factor and how much was either excessive or too little because we didn't understand the connection between the two. So that then made us go back and start thinking about more intently the medical necessity and capturing the [diagnosis] codes to support the ICD-10 codes . . . because [the payer] didn't define in advance, so we had to retrospectively figure out how we got there.

Interviewer: Got it. So in a way, getting the—it's almost reverse engineering [the payer's] methods from the granular data you were receiving.

Interviewee: That's exactly it, because they didn't define them in advance. So we had to retrospectively figure out how we got [our score].

—administrative leader of a medium-sized single-subspecialty practice

Rather than improving their own understanding of new payment models, some practice leaders decided to delegate their practice's engagement strategy to vendors and consultants. For example, this practice leader delegated decisionmaking in MACRA MIPS to an EHR vendor:

> Our EHR is the one that basically does MACRA for us. So in the licensing terms that we have with our EHR, [the vendor] is the one that basically runs the reports, submits the data for MACRA, all that kind of stuff. It tells us, basically, what the new measurements are going to be, what packages that they have to assist the doctors and meeting those measurements and whether we're interested or not—you know, that type of sort of thing. I've done MACRA research on my own just to get prepared but it hasn't been in-depth, again because [EHR vendor] is the one who does everything for us.
>
> —office manager of a medium-sized single-subspecialty practice

Strategies Enabled by Understanding Complex Payment Models

Some practices were able to succeed in complex new payment models by exploiting their detailed understanding of them. These practices ensured that they got credit for the quality of care they already delivered, rather than attempting to make changes in patient care. One approach to this was to thoroughly capture the diagnostic codes that serve as the basis for case-mix adjustment for cost and quality outcomes measures:

> It's extracting the codes that those words [in physicians' notes] represent then putting them on the billing statement, that's what the insurance companies and CMS need to see. So what we've ultimately done, I think, is just make sure that what they say and do is captured. Which would, I guess, imply that we haven't really changed anything except our effectiveness in reporting to show that the quality's improved.
>
> —administrative leader of a medium-sized single-subspecialty practice

Some practices modified their EHR user interfaces to prompt physicians to enter diagnostic codes, thus ensuring that they were thoroughly capturing these codes. Other practices hired scribes, employed a dedicated coding staff that prompted physicians to modify their bills before submitting them, or used natural language processing to identify unbilled diagnoses. Once diagnoses were thoroughly captured, some practices said that they preferred cost and outcomes measures from the menu offered by MACRA MIPS. These measures are risk-adjusted, so thorough coding was expected to lead to high performance ratings, whereas process measures (e.g., whether patients received screening services), which are not risk-adjusted and on which most practices perform well, could limit the opportunity to be a high-performing outlier.

Actively managing patient attribution was another strategy that practices used to improve their performance ratings, especially on measures of costs of care. By taking steps to attribute the highest-cost patients away from the practice (without interrupting patient-physician relationships or denying care), a practice could *improve* its performance in certain shared savings models:

> One of the things that we did early in the ACOs was off-load the cost of skilled nursing care. It's almost always the primary care physician that's responsible for that if that person is also in the ACO. All of the costs for the [most expensive] patients, even with a high risk-adjustment factor, are saddled back to the ACO. . . . [Savings seemed to come from] people

managing the cost of nursing home care better, and that's why they stayed in the green, the shared savings. What they are kind of missing is that most of that occurred because somebody created a separate tax ID for the work in the nursing home so that it didn't impact the ACO. Didn't change cost structure. Didn't change the acuity of the patient. It just subtracted that ugly cost from the ACO.

—leader of MSSP ACO

Similar attribution considerations could shape multispecialty practices' strategies for the QPP. For example, one such practice included its primary care physicians in an AAPM (where they bore financial risk on costs of care) but placed its subspecialists in MIPS (where they did not bear such risk). This arrangement was described as advantageous because the practice's primary care patients were not especially high-risk. However, many of the patients who only saw the practice's subspecialists were very high-risk and would be attributed to the practice if they lacked outside primary care physicians—which occurred frequently enough to create an unfavorable AAPM risk profile, despite risk adjustment. In another example, a single-specialty practice referred complex patients who lacked primary care physicians to local generalists. In addition to describing these referrals as being good medicine (because these complex patients benefited from having primary care), even a single visit to a primary care physician would attribute the patient away from the subspecialty group under MIPS attribution rules, even if the patient saw his or her subspecialist more frequently.

New Findings: More Prominent Risk Aversion Among Physician Practices

Overview of Findings

Despite general enthusiasm for APMs that involved bonuses, practices that spanned multiple specialties and markets reported a high degree of financial risk aversion, which influenced their decisions to engage in new payment models. These practices sought either to avoid downside risk or off-load it to partners (e.g., hospitals and device manufacturers) whenever possible.

For smaller practices, taking on debt to finance the infrastructure investments that were necessary to succeed in APMs represented another form of financial risk. These practices were attracted to APMs that offered subsidies for up-front infrastructure investments and to partners that provided such infrastructure at nominal cost, in exchange for a share of any bonuses received. Some larger practices—especially those with prior experience taking losses in APMs—renegotiated their contracts to shift more risk back to payers.

Detailed Findings

Increasing Risk Aversion Affected Practices' Decisions to Participate in APMs

In our 2014 study, several participants across study markets expressed enthusiasm for participating in new APMs that included downside risk. Take, for example, this physician leader who had not yet participated in an APM, but who looked forward to a change from FFS:

> As we look forward to value-based payments, we couldn't be more excited. It speaks to all of our strengths. . . . There's enough money in the entire system here such that, if we can now migrate away from incentives that incent providers economically based upon how much of something they do . . . but we can now focus them more on saying, . . . "You're achieving these quality scores; you're achieving this kind of quality and this kind of patient satisfaction . . . and if you're doing it for less, then there's no reason why you should not benefit from that." . . . I absolutely love that.
> —physician leader, medium-sized single-subspecialty practice

In 2018, however, enthusiasm for APMs involving downside risk was relatively rare; physician practices and provider systems were generally risk averse—in some cases due to experiences with risk-based contracting over the past several years. Practices tended to prefer APMs with little or no downside risk—such as PFP and one-sided, upside-only shared savings models.

At the same time, there was widespread consensus that practices eventually will be compelled into higher-risk contracting mechanisms, either through regulatory requirements or the continuing erosion in FFS-based payment rates. Consequently, a range of practices admitted to "tiptoeing" into, or moderating the growth of, their high-risk contracting until they are able to develop the clinical and business infrastructure necessary to manage the risk and perform well under these models.

However, even certain practices that had relied until recently on capitated payment, or had built up extensive care management infrastructures, were wary of taking on additional downside risk. To a certain extent, this reluctance was a product of financial uncertainties created by having to manage mixed portfolios of value-based and FFS-based payment models in certain markets; but it was also partly a result of higher weighting of downside—compared to upside—risk in specific value-based models.

Low Tolerance for Risk

A number of physicians and practice leaders across community sites reported having a low tolerance for risk, particularly if they did not have previous experience with contracts involving downside risk (i.e., requiring the practice to cover financial losses from the model) or the infrastructure to manage patients under these models:

> I think the key [with taking on downside risk], and it's again something we don't have any experience in, would be having the stop-loss insurance to cover the downside risk adequately so that nobody would have to write a check, because that's where the stress comes from.
> —physician leader of large multispecialty practice

> We're an MSSP Track 1. We debated hard about going MSSP Track 1+, and just felt like our infrastructure is not equipped yet to really take on risk comfortably. But we will definitely reevaluate that going into the future.
> —practice leader of large multispecialty practice

Even practices that already had a well-developed care management infrastructure said that they avoided payment models with downside risks, based on calculations of the potential upside bonus versus the potential downside penalty. The risk trade-off described by one interviewee not only illustrates this calculation but also predicts being compelled to accept such trade-offs in the future:

> We did an upside only, an MSSP Track 1. We didn't take a risk contract. . . . [W]e did an operating analysis and felt like we had the systems in place so we could handle it. But when we did the financial analysis, and we looked at the shared savings and the shared risk models, the shared risk models offered very little additional upside, but the downside was dramatic . . . and we just said for $2 million more, we're not willing to take $17 million [potential] hit, right? So it just didn't make sense. Now CMS is going to—they're going to force the hand.
> —administrative leader of large multispecialty practice

A low tolerance for risk appears to have persisted—despite the substantial trend toward mergers, formation of ACOs, clinical networks, and other forms of consolidation among providers—because organizations were apprehensive about the possibility of absorbing an income reduction:

[Since 2014], there's been a lot more physician practices being acquired by hospital corporations and physicians becoming employees of those organizations. There's also been a trend of physicians in facilities partnering more to create either accountable care organizations . . . [or] what I'll call a clinically integrated network, where they are trying to position themselves more as an organized group to the market. But in spite of those moves, the marketplace in general is still pretty risk-averse. Physician organizations are willing to talk to carriers about entering into arrangements where they will try and work to reduce medical spend and have abilities to earn bonuses, but they don't want to take any risk and lose anything if they don't perform well. . . . The baseline is, "I can't make less than I did last year." I would say it's mostly with physician organizations. [But] hospitals also really aren't taking any risks for anything right now.

—health plan leader

Risk Aversion Guided Practices' Strategies Within New Payment Models

Risk aversion guided practices' decisions not only on which payment models to participate in but also on how to respond to new payment models. Even as practices transitioned from fee-for-service to APM models, they sought to off-load downside financial risk onto partners (in exchange for reduced bonuses) to avoid taking on debt to fund infrastructure improvements necessary to succeed in APMs and to limit the likelihood of internal blowback among their physicians when their incentives changed.

Strategy: Off-Loading Risk onto Partners

Some practices sought out specific strategic partnerships as a way to mitigate risk. For example, one specialty practice planned to participate in a new bundled payment program, but only because they were able to partner with a "convener" who would absorb the downside risk, which the practice otherwise would not have accepted on its own:

> We're looking at BPCI-A, the advanced version. . . . So [hospital and device manufacturers] have been doing bundled payment stuff as a facilitator or convener for a long time. We got what seemed like reasonable proposals from both of them. The [device manufacturer] one, for example, they'll take all the downside risk, and they want a 30 percent cut of the upside. So okay, that seems reasonable, since we're getting into stuff that we don't know . . . and wouldn't be doing on our own. So if it's a downside, it's their problem; if it's an upside, it's found money for us.
>
> —physician leader of small orthopedic practice

Other practices partnered with hospitals to limit their exposure to downside risk, as in the case of this primary care practice's involvement in a local commercial ACO:

> [Commercial payer] has a value-based incentive right now, . . . and it's a matter of, "Well, how are you doing on measuring colonoscopies and different metrics like that?" The payment's not very big, but there's no risk to it and it's already stuff we're doing, you know. . . . [Local hospital] here has what they call a physician partnership. Right now there is no downside to it. . . . They do have an ACO part, but we are in just the partnership. . . . We'll agree to be in this to measure our metrics and we do get payments from that. Like I said, they're small, but there's no downside to it. It's just a matter of reporting to them.
>
> —practicing physician in a small primary care practice

Another market observer predicted that expanding APMs, coupled with physicians' general aversion to downside risk, would create opportunities for private equity investors, who are accustomed to such risk, to co-own and co-manage physician practices:

> So ACOs, in general, I think they're probably going to convert to investors coming in, recognizing that if they've got a Medicare Advantage plan with all these patients, I don't know that the physicians will be willing to take the risk sufficiently to be in charge of that, although they should. It's going to be another boom for the business guys that get it and understand that the physicians need to help manage it. . . . They'll give physicians ownership and incentive to be engaged, but the business guys are going to get most of the money. . . . I don't even think it's that [physicians] won't have the money, . . . they've got the money to establish this, but it means that they've got a risk on the downside if it doesn't perform well. [A]nd they know too well how fragile that can be if you have physicians coming in that are either not paying attention or sufficiently managed or incentivized.
> —administrative leader of an ACO

Strategy: Avoiding Infrastructure Improvement Debt

Practices' strategies for succeeding in APMs frequently involved investing in new or upgraded patient care capabilities. But even in APMs that lacked explicit downside penalties, this type of investment, when financed by loans, could create financial risk if bonuses failed to materialize when expected. This financial risk could be especially significant for small, independent practices lacking access to low-cost credit. Such practices were therefore attracted to APMs that subsidized infrastructure investments up front, such as Medicare's CPC+ program:

> A program that we think has been extremely successful is [Medicare's] Comprehensive Primary Care Plus program, CPC+. . . . They actually pay you a lot to put in infrastructure, so they're funding a lot of your medical home costs and a lot of your advance payment costs, because you meet the criteria and were accepted [into the program] . . . and then there's significant payment increases that you get in bonuses for hitting the different targets. And so it's both infrastructure payment and then physician revenue payment, and it's definitely significantly better than what [local commercial plan] does . . . CPC+, I believe, is a significant benefit in regards to value-based payment and physician alignment. And many independent physicians across Michigan and Ohio also got CPC+ designation, and so it helps the physician in practice who's independent get that funding for infrastructure.
> —physician leader of a large multispecialty practice

Other practices were attracted to vendors that provided new capabilities at up-front low cost, again, in exchange for a share of any APM bonuses received. One practice leader described participating in a one-sided ACO model, noting the benefits of working with such a vendor:

> What we liked about [vendor] is that there is no large fee up front. . . . They help us take a look at cost overall . . . get all the claims from Medicare, and they have a good website and app that we use to see, all right, per patient what are our high-risk codes, high-risk diagnosis that we didn't know this patient had because they may have a specialist somewhere that does not send us any notes. . . . So they fill in the blanks on a lot of our information as far as overall patient care . . . and gave us a lot more information to work with. Their model is, we pay very little every year, but whenever shared savings comes in they get a percentage.
> —practicing physician in a small primary care practice

Strategy: Shifting Risk Back to Payers

Among practices that were large enough to renegotiate their risk contracts with payers, some described shifting certain categories of risk back to the payer. Costs that were outside the practice's control—but not outside the payer's control—were the top priorities, especially when practices had already absorbed APM penalties. For example, this large practice negotiated greater protection from losses due to escalating pharmaceutical costs, in exchange for reductions in possible bonuses:

> If you can cure hepatitis C, and there's a cohort of tens of thousands of people out there with hepatitis C, you're not seriously going to ask us to withhold those drugs, because we're not going to. That's unethical. And yet you will hold us accountable for the cost of those drugs. So, let me get this right, and this is what happened two years ago, is Sovaldi, we lost in our commercial contracts because of Sovaldi, we paid penalties to the commercial payers who had to purchase those drugs, right? So, we are then paying pharma for their price escalations. . . . [But] the payers are negotiating with pharma, right? So that's just wrong. That is just completely wrong. Makes us furious. We have negotiated, we have made it clear how we feel about this and that is definitely not risk we should be taking on. . . . [Now] we have some protection. It's some complicated thing, which is sort of a retrospective if certain price trends hit certain thresholds . . . we don't pay a penalty, but we don't get any of the shared savings [if we save on drugs].
>
> —physician leader of large multispecialty practice, regarding
> a shared savings payment model

Conclusions

Four years later, the primary findings of our 2014 study concerning the effects of APMs on physician practices persist. Across markets and specialties, there were practices of all sizes that took advantage of APMs by developing new capabilities (e.g., to provide better behavioral health care or to more effectively manage population health) intended to improve patient care, adopting new models of care (e.g., care outside of office visits), managing data (e.g., investing in health information exchanges to more quickly identify and assist high-needs patients), and engaging with new partners (e.g., by joining ACOs or working with hospitals in bundled payment models). As in 2014, practices in the current study also served as buffers between payers and individual physicians by modifying or completely absorbing financial incentives rather than passing them directly to frontline clinicians. Again, practices that faced penalties and rewards based on costs of care rarely constructed cost-based financial incentives for their individual physicians, often opting instead to transmit incentives based on quality measures.

The challenges of APMs that we observed in 2014 also persisted. The data necessary to perform well in APMs were frequently incomplete or difficult for practices to analyze. Data lags continued to be particularly problematic. Even data elements as critical as patient lists and performance targets in APMs with substantial downside risk continued to reach practices well into the payment year and were sometimes even changed mid-year. In some cases, unintentional operational errors identified in 2014 remained uncorrected in 2018, resulting in nonpayment of earned bonuses and discouragement of practice leadership regarding participation in future APMs. Many practices reported ongoing tension between FFS and APM incentives simultaneously received from different payers—or even from the same payer when an APM led to opposing financial incentives within the same practice (e.g., in shared savings models involving both primary care and subspecialist physicians). Nearly all practices continued to be challenged by the cacophony of measures they received from payers, which many described as worsening under the MACRA QPP.

Our current study also identified three sets of findings that were new or more prominent in 2018 than in 2014. First, practices described an accelerating pace of change in APMs. Physician practices, health systems, and even the consultants advising them on APMs had trouble keeping up with the proliferation of new models, with some calling for a "time out" to allow them to better adapt to current APMs before entering new ones. Unanticipated reversals in payment models were particularly challenging because they interfered with practices' ability to enjoy a return on APM-driven investments, and they interrupted formation of new partnerships. These unpredictable, sudden reversals in government payment programs accompanied changes of administration at both the state and federal levels. The political aspect of these changes seemed like a new intrusion into a previously technical area of government policy, where program performance rather than ideology has long been the basis of decisionmaking. As one market observer remarked, this new unpredictability of government programs increased the importance of private sector APMs, which could help stabilize practices' incentives.

Second, practices and market observers reported that APMs had become more complex since 2014. For instance, the QPP, with its many decisions concerning program participation and measure selection, was an exemplar of APM complexity. However, our respondents cited many instances of APM complexity from private and state-level payers as well. Multiple leaders of practices across markets, specialties, and sizes described struggling to understand complex APMs sponsored by both government and private payers. Some practices exerted great effort to analyze the mechanics of payment models and simulate expected financial returns from incentives (to the point of reverse-engineering incentive programs based on available information)—but this approach was out-of-reach for small practices with limited investment resources. Others placed their trust in vendors, for example, by relying on their EHR vendors to "do MACRA for us." A relatively small number of practices reported understanding complex APMs in detail. These practices were medium to large in size, and they reported having invested extensively in internal analytic capabilities. Such practices were able to use their knowledge to pursue novel strategies—beyond the complete capture of comorbidities (i.e., attending to risk adjustment) reported in 2014—to earn bonuses, sometimes without materially changing patient care. These strategies included actively managing patient attribution and strategically choosing risk-adjusted outcomes and cost measures that would reward complete comorbidity capture.

Third, practices reported greater risk aversion in 2018 than they did in 2014, when a general enthusiasm for "taking risk" was more widespread. Practice leaders—some of whom reported experiencing substantial losses in APMs since 2014—sought to avoid or off-load downside risk to partners, often in exchange for reduced upside bonus prospects. For smaller practices, making up-front investment in the capabilities encouraged or required by APMs was a substantial source of downside risk; accordingly, these practices reported preferring models and partners that defrayed these up-front costs in exchange for reduced bonus potential. These findings are consistent with a prior survey of 82 ACOs in MSSP Track 1, in which 71 percent of ACO leaders reported that they would likely leave MSSP if forced to accept more downside risk (Dickson 2018b).

Despite these challenges, physicians and physician practice leaders remained enthusiastic about APMs in principle, especially when they saw new payment models as enabling improvements in patient care. Even in practices that had incurred penalties or not received earned bonuses due to operational errors, some leaders reported that these care improvements made their engagement in APMs worthwhile.

Implications

While our study was qualitative, descriptive, and sampled for diversity rather than representativeness, the detailed data we gathered spanned six markets and a diversity of physician practice types, with corroboration from other market observers. The persistence of findings from our 2014 study, such as barriers stemming from data availability and program execution, suggests that these problems cannot be solved quickly or easily. Sustained efforts are probably necessary to identify such barriers and support physician practices' efforts to engage with APMs, with the ultimate goal of improving patient care.

Our findings also have the following new implications for practices, payers, and other stakeholders:

Simpler APMs Might Help Practices Focus on Improving Patient Care

The complexity of new APMs has confused some physician practice leaders, disengaged others, and induced a smaller set of practices to make substantial investments just to understand these APMs in detail. When practices do not understand APMs, they are unsure of whether to invest in performance improvement, or how to do so in ways that will be rewarded or reimbursed by these new programs—regardless of whether APMs involve downside risk. When practices understand APMs well, they are able to find ways to succeed (and substantially outperform other practices on APM performance measures), but without necessarily changing patient care (e.g., through strategies that affect patient attribution), especially when practice leaders believe their quality is already high. Our findings suggest that the greater the complexity of APMs, the greater the potential financial return on practices' investments in understanding them. Simplifying APMs might help tip the balance back toward improving patient care as the preferred strategy for earning financial rewards.

Practices Would Benefit from a Stable, Predictable, Moderately Paced Pathway for APMs

The accelerating pace of change in APMs has exhausted not only physician practices but also the consultants advising them. Worse, unanticipated reversals in payment policies have prevented practices from recovering the costs and reaping the rewards of their substantial APM-driven investments in care improvement. A slower, more predictable pace of change in payment models seems likely to benefit practices, payers, and other stakeholders. Practices might consider negotiating longer-term contracts with payers, with built-in penalties for early unilateral termination of the model (or for substantial deviation from the prespecified course of change). To insulate APMs from the vagaries of electoral politics, efforts that involve private-sector payers might prove more stable over time.

Practices Need New Capabilities and Timely Data to Succeed in APMs

As in 2014, many physician practices in our current study—especially small, independent practices—reported that they lacked the internal skills and experience necessary to perform well in APMs. Data management and analysis were seen as critical skills; but without timely, complete, and accurate performance data, even practices with well-developed data infrastructures were unable to assess their improvement efforts, make course corrections, or even know their positions relative to performance targets. Helping practices invest in these skill sets and supplying them with timely, understandable performance data will likely be a critical contribution to the ultimate successfulness of many APMs. Conversely, payment models that are poorly executed (e.g., with serious, persistent operational errors) and unsupportive of physician practices could undermine future engagement in APMs, not to mention fail to improve care.

Reducing Practices' Access to Upside-Only APMs Risks Disengaging Them

In our current study, physician practices expressed increasing aversion to downside risk in APMs (regardless of APM complexity). With the exception of larger practices that had extensive experience in managed care, practices generally sought upside-only APMs. When faced with APMs that featured downside risk, practices took steps to off-load this risk to partners. Given this risk aversion, and given the likelihood that practices will find ways to minimize downside risk in any event, payers should carefully weigh the anticipated advantages and disadvantages of mandating APMs with downside risk. In some cases, continuing to offer upside-only APMs or finding other ways to help practices manage downside risk (e.g., subsidizing up-front investments in new practice capabilities) might improve APM uptake—especially among practices with limited experience in risk contracts.

Designing APMs to Encourage Clinical Changes That Individual Physicians See as Valuable Might Improve Their Effectiveness

As in 2014, physicians were broadly supportive of APMs that enabled their practices to make noticeable improvements in patient care. In such cases, physicians reported intrinsic satisfaction with clinical improvements, sometimes even when these improvements did not result in financial bonuses. However, when APMs' principal impact on physicians was to create new documentation and reporting burdens—or there was no perceptible improvement in patient care—physicians generally reported disengagement and skepticism that anything had improved, even when they received bonuses. Co-designing APMs with practicing physicians and other leaders of their practices might help improve physician engagement and the chances that APMs will produce real improvements in patient care.

Bibliography

Abrahamson, K., E. Miech, H. W. Davila, C. Mueller, V. Cooke, and G. Arling, "Pay-for-Performance Policy and Data-Driven Decision Making Within Nursing Homes: A Qualitative Study," *BMJ Quality & Safety*, Vol. 24, No. 5, 2015, pp. 311–317.

Addicott, R., and S. M. Shortell, "How 'Accountable' Are Accountable Care Organizations?" *Health Care Management Review*, Vol. 39, No. 4, 2014, pp. 270–278.

Afendulis, C. C., L. A. Hatfield, B. E. Landon, J. Gruber, M. B. Landrum, R. E. Mechanic, D. E. Zinner, and M. E. Chernew, "Early Impact of Carefirst's Patient-Centered Medical Home with Strong Financial Incentives," *Health Affairs (Millwood)*, Vol. 36, No. 3, 2017, pp. 468–475.

Albanese, N. P., A. M. Pignato, and S. V. Monte, "Provider Perception of Pharmacy Services in the Patient-Centered Medical Home," *Journal of Pharmacy Practice*, Vol. 30, No. 6, 2017, pp. 612–620.

Alidina, S., E. C. Schneider, S. J. Singer, and M. B. Rosenthal, "Structural Capabilities in Small and Medium-Sized Patient-Centered Medical Homes," *American Journal of Managed Care*, Vol. 20, No. 7, 2014, pp. E265–277.

Allen-Dicker, J., S. J. Herzig, and R. Kerbel, "Global Payment Contract Attitudes and Comprehension Among Internal Medicine Physicians," *American Journal of Managed Care*, Vol. 21, No. 8, 2015, pp. E474–479.

Alpert, A., H. Hsi, and M. Jacobson, "Evaluating the Role of Payment Policy in Driving Vertical Integration in the Oncology Market," *Health Affairs (Millwood)*, Vol. 36, No. 4, 2017, pp. 680–688.

Althausen, P. L., and L. Mead, "Bundled Payments for Care Improvement: Lessons Learned in the First Year, *Journal of Orthopaedic Trauma*, Vol. 30, Suppl. 5, 2016, pp. S50–S53.

Anderson, A. C., E. O'Rourke, M. H. Chin, N. A. Ponce, S. M. Bernheim, and H. Burstin, "Promoting Health Equity and Eliminating Disparities Through Performance Measurement and Payment," *Health Affairs (Millwood)*, Vol. 37, No. 3, 2018, pp. 371–377.

Angier, H., J. P. O'Malley, M. Marino, K. J. McConnell, E. Cottrell, R. L. Jacob, S. Likumahuwa-Ackman, J. Heintzman, N. Huguet, S. R. Bailey, and J. E. Devoe, "Evaluating Community Health Centers' Adoption of a New Global Capitation Payment (Echange) Study Protocol," *Contemporary Clinical Trials*, Vol. 52, 2017, pp. 35–38.

Arnold, M. E., L. Buys, and F. Fullas, "Impact of Pharmacist Intervention in Conjunction with Outpatient Physician Follow-Up Visits After Hospital Discharge On Readmission Rate," *American Journal of Health-System Pharmacy*, Vol. 72, No. 11, Suppl. 1, 2015, pp. S36–S42.

ASPE Office of Health Policy, *Individual Market Premium Changes: 2013–2017*, ASPE Data Point, Washington, D.C.: Department of Health and Human Services, 2017.

Balasubramanian, B. A., M. Marino, D. J. Cohen, R. L. Ward, A. Preston, R. J. Springer, S. R. Lindner, S. Edwards, K. J. McConnell, B. F. Crabtree, W. L. Miller, K. C. Stange, and L. I. Solberg, "Use of Quality Improvement Strategies Among Small to Medium-Size US Primary Care Practices," *Annals of Family Medicine*, Vol. 16, Suppl. 1, 2018, pp. S35–S43.

Baloh, J., A. C. MacKinney, K. J. Mueller, T. Vaughn, X. Zhu, and F. Ullrich, "Developmental Strategies and Challenges of Rural Accountable Care Organizations," *Rural Policy Brief*, Vol. 3, 2015, pp. 1–4.

Barnes, A. J., L. Unruh, A. Chukmaitov, and E. Van Ginneken, "Accountable Care Organizations in the USA: Types, Developments and Challenges," *Health Policy*, Vol. 118, No. 1, 2014, pp. 1–7.

Barr, S. M., and M. L. Mattioli, "Accountable Care and Integration: A Challenge for Credentialing and Risk Management," *Journal of Healthcare Risk Management*, Vol. 34, No. 1, 2014, pp. 28–36.

Basu, S., R. S. Phillips, Z. Song, A. Bitton, and B. E. Landon, "High Levels of Capitation Payments Needed to Shift Primary Care Toward Proactive Team and Nonvisit Care," *Health Affairs (Millwood)*, Vol. 36, No. 9, 2017, pp. 1599–1605.

Bazzoli, G. J., M. P. Thompson, and T. M. Waters, "Medicare Payment Penalties and Safety Net Hospital Profitability: Minimal Impact on These Vulnerable Hospitals," *Health Services Research*, February 8, 2018.

Beaulieu-Volk, D. "Will Concierge Medicine Become Mainstream?" *FiercePracticeManagement*, January 23, 2015a. As of September 19, 2018:
https://www.fiercehealthcare.com/practices/will-concierge-medicine-become-mainstream

———, "Concentrated Concierge Practices: Too Much of a Good Thing?" *FiercePracticeManagement*, May 5, 2015b. As of September 19, 2018:
https://www.fiercehealthcare.com/practices/concentrated-concierge-practices-too-much-a-good-thing

Bendix, J., "Reinventing Primary Care (Cover Story)," *Medical Economics*, Vol. 92, No. 12, 2015, pp. 20–24.

Benzer, J. K., G. J. Young, J. F. Burgess, Jr., E. Baker, D. C. Mohr, M. P. Charns, and P. J. Kaboli, "Sustainability of Quality Improvement Following Removal of Pay-for-Performance Incentives," *Journal of General Internal Medicine*, Vol. 29, No. 1, 2014, pp. 127–132.

Berenson, R., "Addressing Pricing Power in Integrated Delivery: The Limits of Antitrust," *Journal of Health Politics, Policy and Law*, Vol. 40, No. 4, 2015, pp. 711–744.

Blackstone, E. A., and J. P. Fuhr, Jr., "The Economics of Medicare Accountable Care Organizations," *American Health & Drug Benefits*, Vol. 9, No. 1, 2016, pp. 11–19.

Blewett, L. A., D. Spencer, and P. Huckfeldt, "Minnesota Integrated Health Partnership Demonstration: Implementation of a Medicaid ACO Model," *Journal of Health Politics, Policy and Law*, Vol. 42, No. 6, 2017, pp. 1127–1142.

Bolz, N. J., and R. Iorio, "Bundled Payments: Our Experience at an Academic Medical Center," *Journal of Arthroplasty*, Vol. 31, No. 5, 2016, pp. 932–935.

Bradley, E. H., L. A. Curry, and K. J. Devers, "Qualitative Data Analysis for Health Services Research: Developing Taxonomy, Themes, and Theory," *Health Services Research*, Vol. 42, No. 4, 2007, pp. 1758–1772.

Brosig-Koch, J., H. Hennig-Schmidt, N. Kairies-Schwarz, and D. Wiesen, "The Effects of Introducing Mixed Payment Systems for Physicians: Experimental Evidence," *Health Economics*, Vol. 26, No. 2, 2017, pp. 243–262.

Carey, K., and M. Y. Lin, "Readmissions to New York Hospitals Fell for Three Target Conditions from 2008 to 2012, Consistent with Medicare Goals," *Health Affairs (Millwood)*, Vol. 34, No. 6, 2015, pp. 978–985.

Carrillo, J. E., V. A. Carrillo, R. Guimento, J. Mucaria, and J. Leiman, "The New York-Presbyterian Regional Health Collaborative: A Three-Year Progress Report," *Health Affairs (Millwood)*, Vol. 33, No. 11, 2014, pp. 1985–1992.

Castellucci, M., "Most Medicare ACOs Still Risk-Averse," *Modern Healthcare*, Vol. 47, No. 45, 2017a. As of October 11, 2018:
https://www.pressreader.com/usa/modern-healthcare/20171106/281758449557359

———, "Providers Want the CMS to Create Alternative Pay Models That Are More Flexible," *Modern Healthcare*, Vol. 47, No. 47, 2017b. As of October 11, 2018:
https://www.pressreader.com/usa/modern-healthcare/20171127/281625305613644

———, "To Stay Independent, Physicians Turn to ACOs," *Modern Healthcare*, Vol. 48, No. 6, 2018a. As of October 11, 2018:
https://www.acponline.org/system/files/documents/about_acp/chapters/ga/to_stay_independent.pdf

———, "CMS Next Generation ACO Changes Prompt Early Exits, Potential Lawsuit," *Modern Healthcare*, Vol. 48, No. 13, 2018. As of October 11, 2018:
http://www.modernhealthcare.com/article/20180322/NEWS/180329958

Cen, X., H. Temkin-Greener, and Y. Li, "Medicare Bundled Payments for Post-Acute Care: Characteristics and Baseline Performance of Participating Skilled Nursing Facilities," *Medical Care Research and Review*, April 1, 2018 [epub ahead of print].

Centers for Medicare and Medicaid Services, "Bundled Payments for Care Improvement Initiative (BPCI): Fact Sheet," April 18, 2016. As of June 15, 2018:
https://www.cms.gov/newsroom/fact-sheets/bundled-payments-care-improvement-initiative-bpci-fact-sheet

————, "Bundled Payments for Care Improvement (BPCI) Initiative: General Information," May 7, 2018. As of June 15, 2018:
https://innovation.cms.gov/initiatives/bundled-payments

————,"Comprehensive Care for Joint Replacement Model," June 15, 2018. As of September 12, 2018:
https://innovation.cms.gov/initiatives/cjr

Chen, B., and V. Y. Fan, "Global Budget Payment: Proposing the CAP Framework," *Inquiry*, Vol. 53, 2016.

Chen, C. T., D. C. Ackerly, and G. Gottlieb, "Transforming Healthcare Delivery: Why and How Accountable Care Organizations Must Evolve," *Journal of Hospital Medicine*, Vol. 11, No. 9, 2016, pp. 658–661.

Cole, E. S., C. Campbell, M. L. Diana, L. Webber, and R. Culbertson, "Patient-Centered Medical Homes in Louisiana Had Minimal Impact on Medicaid Population's Use of Acute Care and Costs," *Health Affairs (Millwood)*, Vol. 34, No. 1, 2015, pp. 87–94.

Colla, C. H., V. A. Lewis, S. L. Bergquist, and S. M. Shortell, "Accountability Across the Continuum: The Participation of Postacute Care Providers in Accountable Care Organizations," *Health Services Research*, Vol. 51, No. 4, 2016, pp. 1595–1611.

Colla, C. H., V. A. Lewis, S. M. Shortell, and E. S. Fisher, "First National Survey of ACOs Finds That Physicians Are Playing Strong Leadership and Ownership Roles," *Health Affairs (Millwood)*, Vol. 33, No. 6, 2014, pp. 964–971.

Colla, C. H., V. A. Lewis, E. Tierney, and D. B. Muhlestein, "Hospitals Participating in ACOs Tend to Be Large and Urban, Allowing Access to Capital and Data," *Health Affairs (Millwood)*, Vol. 35, No. 3, 2016, pp. 431–439.

Colwell, J., "Physicians Chart New Path into Direct Primary Care," *Medical Economics*, Vol. 93, No. 12, 2016, pp. 18–19, 24–26.

Courtney, P. M., D. D. Bohl, E. C. Lau, K. L. Ong, J. J. Jacobs, and C. J. Della Valle, "Risk Adjustment Is Necessary in Medicare Bundled Payment Models for Total Hip and Knee Arthroplasty," *Journal of Arthroplasty*, Vol. 33, No. 8, 2018, pp. 2368–2375.

Crosson, F. J., K. Bloniarz, D. Glass, and J. Mathews, "Medpac's Urgent Recommendation: Eliminate MIPS, Take a Different Direction," *Health Affairs Blog*, March 16, 2018. As of September 19, 2018:
https://www.healthaffairs.org/do/10.1377/hblog20180309.302220/full/

Cuccia, T. J., "Practice Acquisitions: What Physicians Need to Know," *Medical Economics*, Vol. 91, No. 14, 2014, pp. 21–24.

D'Aunno, T., L. Broffman, M. Sparer, and S. R. Kumar, "Factors That Distinguish High-Performing Accountable Care Organizations in the Medicare Shared Savings Program," *Health Services Research*, Vol. 53, No. 1, 2016, pp. 120–137.

da Graca, B., G. O. Ogola, C. Fullerton, R. McCorkle, and N. S. Fleming, "Offsetting Patient-Centered Medical Homes Investment Costs Through Per-Member-Per-Month Or Medicare Merit-Based Incentive Payment System Incentive Payments," *Journal of Ambulatory Care Management*, Vol. 41, No. 2, 2018, pp. 105–113.

Dickson, V., "Providers Want Overhaul of Medicare Hip, Knee Payment Test," *Modern Healthcare*, Vol. 45, No. 37, 2015. As of October 11, 2018:
https://www.pressreader.com/usa/modern-healthcare/20150914/281681138659568

————, "Providers Urge Expanded Use of Multipayer Care Delivery Models," *Modern Healthcare*, Vol. 47, No. 38, 2017. As of October 11, 2018:
https://www.pressreader.com/usa/modern-healthcare/20170918/281694024950417

————, "CMS Meets MIPS Reporting Goals, But Thousands of Doctors Still Face Penalties," *Modern Healthcare*, Vol. 48, No. 23, 2018a. As of October 11, 2018:
http://www.modernhealthcare.com/article/20180531/NEWS/180539986

———, "Heading for the Exit: Rather Than Face Risk, Many ACOs Could Leave," *Modern Healthcare*, May 12, 2018b. As of September 19, 2018:
http://www.modernhealthcare.com/article/20180512/news/180519966

———, "Doctors Urge Congress to Eliminate MACRA Opt-Out Policy," *Modern Healthcare*, June 5, 2018c. As of September 19, 2018:
http://www.modernhealthcare.com/article/20180605/news/180609960

———, "MIPS on Track to Be SGR 2.0 If Not Fixed, Doctors Say," *Modern Healthcare*, July 26, 2018d. As of September 19, 2018:
http://www.modernhealthcare.com/article/20180726/news/180729931

Dickson, V., S. Muchmore, and S. Livingston, "Final MACRA Rule Expands Exemptions, Flexibility," *Modern Healthcare*, Vol. 46, No. 42, 2016. As of October 11, 2018:
http://www.modernhealthcare.com/article/20161014/NEWS/161019942

Doherty, R., "Assessing the Patient Care Implications of 'Concierge' and Other Direct Patient Contracting Practices: A Policy Position Paper from the American College of Physicians," *Annals of Internal Medicine*, Vol. 163, No. 12, 2015, pp. 949–952.

Douven, R., T. G. McGuire, and J. M. McWilliams, "Avoiding Unintended Incentives in ACO Payment Models," *Health Affairs (Millwood)*, Vol. 34, No. 1, 2015, pp. 143–149.

Driessen, J., and T. West, "Recent Evidence on the Inclusion of Hospice and Palliative Care Physicians in Medicare Shared Savings Program Accountable Care Organization Networks," *Journal of Palliative Medicine*, Vol. 21, No. 3, 2017, pp. 373–375.

Driessen, J., and Y. Zhang, "Trends in the Inclusion of Mental Health Providers in Medicare Shared Savings Program ACOs," *Psychiatric Services*, Vol. 68, No. 3, 2017, pp. 303–305.

Edmondson, W. R., "The Per Capita Payment Model," *Journal of Healthcare Management*, Vol. 60, No. 1, 2015, pp. 14–16.

Edwards, S. T., M. K. Abrams, R. J. Baron, R. A. Berenson, E. C. Rich, G. E. Rosenthal, M. B. Rosenthal, and B. E. Landon, "Structuring Payment to Medical Homes After the Affordable Care Act," *Journal of General Internal Medicine*, Vol. 29, No. 10, 2014, pp. 1410–1413.

Edwards, S. T., A. Bitton, J. Hong, and B. E. Landon, "Patient-Centered Medical Home Initiatives Expanded in 2009–13: Providers, Patients, and Payment Incentives Increased," *Health Affairs (Millwood)*, Vol. 33, No. 10, 2014, pp. 1823–1831.

Elbuluk, A. M., and O. R. O'Neill, "Private Bundles: The Nuances of Contracting and Managing Total Joint Arthroplasty Episodes," *Journal of Arthroplasty*, Vol. 32, No. 6, 2017, pp. 1720–1722.

Epstein, A. M., A. K. Jha, E. J. Orav, D. L. Liebman, A. M. Audet, M. A. Zezza, and S. Guterman, "Analysis of Early Accountable Care Organizations Defines Patient, Structural, Cost, and Quality-of-Care Characteristics," *Health Affairs (Millwood)*, Vol. 33, No. 1, 2014, pp. 95–102.

Eskew, P. M., and K. Klink, "Direct Primary Care: Practice Distribution and Cost Across the Nation," *Journal of the American Board of Family Medicine*, Vol. 28, No. 6, 2015, pp. 793–801.

Evans, M., "Many Providers Say No to Bundled-Payment Test," *Modern Healthcare*, Vol. 45, No. 34, 2015a. As of October 11, 2018:
http://www.modernhealthcare.com/article/20150815/MAGAZINE/308159925/many-providers-say-no-to-bundled-payment-test

———, "Primary-Care Docs Reaping the Most from Shared-Savings ACOs," *Modern Healthcare*, Vol. 45, No. 35, 2015b. As of October 11, 2018:
http://www.modernhealthcare.com/article/20150829/MAGAZINE/308299961

Federal Register, Medicare Program; Revisions to Payment Policies Under the Physician Fee Schedule and Other Revisions to Part B for CY 2019; Medicare Shared Savings Program Requirements; Quality Payment Program; and Medicaid Promoting Interoperability Program: A Proposed Rule by the Centers for Medicare & Medicaid Services, July 27, 2018. As of September 19, 2018:
https://www.federalregister.gov/d/2018-14985

Feinstein, D. L., P. Kuhlmann, and P. J. Mucchetti, "Accountable Care Organizations and Antitrust Enforcement: Promoting Competition and Innovation," *Journal of Health Politics, Policy and Law*, Vol. 40, No. 4, 2015, pp. 875–886.

Ferrante, J. M., E. K. Shaw, J. E. Bayly, J. Howard, M. N. Quest, E. C. Clark, and C. Pascal, "Barriers and Facilitators to Expanding Roles of Medical Assistants in Patient-Centered Medical Homes (PCMHs)," *Journal of the American Board of Family Medicine*, Vol. 31, No. 2, 2018, pp. 226–235.

Finkel, E. D., "Why Membership Medicine Is Gaining Physician Attention," *Medical Economics*, Vol. 94, No. 3, 2017, pp. 31–35.

Fiscella, K., and S. H. McDaniel, "The Complexity, Diversity, and Science of Primary Care Teams," *The American Psychologist*, Vol. 73, No. 4, 2018, pp. 451–467.

Fleming, N. S., B. da Graca, G. O. Ogola, S. D. Culler, J. Austin, P. McConnell, R. McCorkle, P. Aponte, M. Massey, and C. Fullerton, "Costs of Transforming Established Primary Care Practices to Patient-Centered Medical Homes (PCMHs)," *Journal of the American Board of Family Medicine*, Vol. 30, No. 4, 2017, pp. 460–471.

Fontaine, P., R. Whitebird, L. I. Solberg, J. Tillema, A. Smithson, and B. F. Crabtree, "Minnesota's Early Experience with Medical Home Implementation: Viewpoints from the Front Lines," *Journal of General Internal Medicine*, Vol. 30, No. 7, 2015, pp. 899–906.

Foote, K. E., and E. E. Varanini, "A Few Thoughts About ACO Antitrust Issues from a Local Enforcement Perspective," *Journal of Health Politics, Policy and Law*, Vol. 40, No. 4, 2015, pp. 887–896.

Friedberg, M. W., P. G. Chen, C. White, O. Jung, L. Raaen, S. Hirshman, E. Hoch, C. Stevens, P. B. Ginsburg, L. P. Casalino, M. Tutty, C. Vargo, and L. Lipinski, *Effects of Health Care Payment Models on Physician Practice in the United States*, Santa Monica, Calif.: RAND Corporation, RR-869-AMA, 2015. As of September 19, 2018: https://www.rand.org/pubs/research_reports/RR869.html

Friedberg, M. W., E. C. Schneider, M. B. Rosenthal, K. G. Volpp, and R. M. Werner, "Association Between Participation in a Multipayer Medical Home Intervention and Changes in Quality, Utilization, and Costs of Care," *JAMA*, Vol. 311, No. 8, 2014, pp. 815–825.

Goldman, R. E., J. Brown, P. Stebbins, D. R. Parker, V. Adewale, R. Shield, M. B. Roberts, C. B. Eaton, and J. M. Borkan, "What Matters in Patient-Centered Medical Home Transformation: Whole System Evaluation Outcomes of the Brown Primary Care Transformation Initiative," *SAGE Open Medicine*, Vol. 6, June 18, 2018 [epub ahead of print].

Grant, L. S., "Demand for Concierge Healthcare Services Is on the Rise," *Journal of Corporate Renewal*, Vol. 29, No. 2, 2016, pp. 24–27.

Gray, C. F., H. A. Prieto, A. T. Duncan, and H. K. Parvataneni, "Arthroplasty Care Redesign Related to the Comprehensive Care for Joint Replacement Model: Results at a Tertiary Academic Medical Center," *Arthroplasty Today*, Vol. 4, No. 2, 2018, pp. 221–226.

Greene, J., "GM Signs Major Health Care Services Deal for Salaried Employees," *Automotive News*, Detroit, Mich.: Crain Communications, 2018.

Greene, J., E. T. Kurtzman, J. H. Hibbard, and V. Overton, "Working Under a Clinic-Level Quality Incentive: Primary Care Clinicians' Perceptions," *Annals of Family Medicine*, Vol. 13, No. 3, 2015, pp. 235–241.

Grogan, C. M., "Encouraging Competition and Cooperation: The Affordable Care Act's Contradiction?" *Journal of Health Politics, Policy and Law*, Vol. 40, No. 4, 2015, pp. 633–638.

Gusmano, M. K., and F. J. Thompson, "An Examination of Medicaid Delivery System Reform Incentive Payment Initiatives Under Way in Six States," *Health Affairs (Millwood)*, Vol. 34, No. 7, 2015, pp. 1162–1169.

Hacker, K., P. Santos, D. Thompson, S. S. Stout, A. Bearse, and R. E. Mechanic, "Early Experience of a Safety Net Provider Reorganizing into an Accountable Care Organization," *Journal of Health Politics, Policy and Law*, Vol. 39, No. 4, 2014, pp. 901–917.

Harris, J. M., I. Elizondo, and A. M. Brown, "Orchestrating ACO Success: How Top Performers Achieve Shared Savings," *Healthcare Financial Management*, Vol. 70, No. 3, 2016, pp. 42–50.

Harrison, M., K. Milbers, T. Mihic, and A. H. Anis, "Incentives in Rheumatology: The Potential Contribution of Physician Responses to Financial Incentives, Public Reporting, and Treatment Guidelines to Health Care Sustainability," *Current Rheumatology Reports*, Vol. 18, No. 7, 2016, p. 42.

Harrod, M., L. E. Weston, C. Robinson, A. Tremblay, C. L. Greenstone, and J. Forman, "'It Goes Beyond Good Camaraderie': A Qualitative Study of the Process of Becoming an Interprofessional Healthcare 'Teamlet,'" *Journal of Interprofessional Care*, Vol. 30, No. 3, 2016, pp. 295–300.

Health Management Technology Magazine, "84% of Med Practices Unclear on MACRA," *Health Management Technology*, February 28, 2017. As of September 19, 2018: https://www.healthmgttech.com/84-med-practices-unclear-macra

Herman, B., "UnitedHealthcare Deal May Spur More Bundled Payments in Cancer Care," *Modern Healthcare*, Vol. 44, No. 51, 2014. As of October 11, 2018: https://www.pressreader.com/usa/modern-healthcare/20141222/281694023129996

Hill, C. E., S. Knox, B. J. Thompson, E. N. Williams, S. A. Hess, and N. Ladany, "Consensual Qualitative Research: An Update," *Journal of Counseling Psychology*, Vol. 52, No. 2, 2005, p. 196.

Himmelstein, D. U., D. Ariely, and S. Woolhandler, "Pay-for-Performance: Toxic to Quality? Insights from Behavioral Economics," *International Journal of Health Services*, Vol. 44, No. 2, 2014, pp. 203–214.

Hing, E., E. Kurtzman, D. T. Lau, C. Taplin, and A. B. Bindman, "Characteristics of Primary Care Physicians in Patient-Centered Medical Home Practices: United States, 2013," *National Health Statistics Reports*, No. 101, 2017, pp. 1–9.

Huff, C., "Direct Primary Care: Concierge Care for the Masses," *Health Affairs (Millwood)*, Vol. 34, No. 12, 2015, pp. 2016–2019.

Humbyrd, C. J., "The Ethics of Bundled Payments in Total Joint Replacement: 'Cherry Picking' and 'Lemon Dropping,'" *Journal of Clinical Ethics*, Vol. 29, No. 1, 2018, pp. 62–68.

Hussain, S. A., C. Arsene, C. Hamstra, T. H. Woehrlen, W. Wiese-Rometsch, and S. R. White, "Successful Resident Engagement in Quality Improvement: The Detroit Medical Center Story," *Journal of Graduate Medical Education*, Vol. 8, No. 2, 2016, pp. 214–218.

Hysong, S. J., R. Sorelle, K. Broussard Smitham, and L. A. Petersen, "Reports of Unintended Consequences of Financial Incentives to Improve Management of Hypertension," *Plos One*, Vol. 12, No. 9, 2017, pp. E0184856.

James, B. C., and G. P. Poulsen, "The Case for Capitation," *Harvard Business Review*, Vol. 94, No. 7–8, 2016, pp. 102–111, 134.

Janus, K., "The Effect of Professional Culture on Intrinsic Motivation Among Physicians in an Academic Medical Center," *Journal of Healthcare Management*, Vol. 59, No. 4, 2014, pp. 287–303; Discussion 303–284.

Johnson, R. M., T. Johnson, S. D. Zimmerman, G. M. Marsh, and O. Garcia-Dominic, "Outcomes of a Seven Practice Pilot in a Pay-for-Performance (P4P)-Based Program in Pennsylvania," *Journal of Racial and Ethnic Health Disparities*, Vol. 2, No. 1, 2015, pp. 139–148.

Johnson, S. R., "Expanding VIP Care," *Modern Healthcare*, Vol. 45, No. 38, 2015, pp. 0020–0020.

Joynt Maddox, K. E., A. P. Sen, L. W. Samson, R. B. Zuckerman, N. Delew, and A. M. Epstein, "Elements of Program Design in Medicare's Value-Based and Alternative Payment Models: A Narrative Review," *Journal of General Internal Medicine*, Vol. 32, No. 11, 2017, pp. 1249–1254.

Kaiser Family Foundation, *Key Facts About the Uninsured Population*, Washington, D.C.: Kaiser Family Foundation, 2017.

Kamath, A. F., P. M. Courtney, K. J. Bozic, S. Mehta, B. S. Parsley, and M. I. Froimson, "Bundled Payment in Total Joint Care: Survey of AAHKS Membership Attitudes and Experience with Alternative Payment Models," *Journal of Arthroplasty*, Vol. 30, No. 12, 2015, pp. 2045–2056.

Kamermayer, A. K., A. R. Leasure, and L. Anderson, "The Effectiveness of Transitions-of-Care Interventions in Reducing Hospital Readmissions and Mortality: A Systematic Review," *Dimensions of Critical Care Nursing*, Vol. 36, No. 6, 2017, pp. 311–316.

Kane, C. K., *Updated Data on Physician Practice Arrangements: Physician Ownership Drops Below 50 Percent*, Chicago, Ill.: American Medical Association, 2017.

Kessell, E., V. Pegany, B. Keolanui, B. D. Fulton, R. M. Scheffler, and S. M. Shortell, "Review of Medicare, Medicaid, and Commercial Quality of Care Measures: Considerations for Assessing Accountable Care Organizations," *Journal of Health Politics, Policy and Law*, Vol. 40, No. 4, 2015, pp. 761–796.

Khazan, O., "Why So Many Insurers Are Leaving Obamacare," *The Atlantic*, May 11, 2017. As of September 19, 2018:
https://www.theatlantic.com/health/archive/2017/05/why-so-many-insurers-are-leaving-obamacare/526137/

Kim, D. H., C. Lloyd, D. K. Fernandez, A. Spielman, and D. Bradshaw, "A Direct Experience in a New Accountable Care Organization: Results, Challenges, and the Role of the Neurosurgeon," *Neurosurgery*, Vol. 80, No. 4s, 2017, pp. S42–S49.

Kleiner, S. A., D. Ludwinski, and W. D. White, "Antitrust and Accountable Care Organizations: Observations for the Physician Market," *Medical Care Research and Review*, Vol. 74, No. 1, 2016, pp. 97–108.

Kocot, S. L. R. White, H. Dajani, C. Garbowski, A. Parry, C. Vargo, C. Botts, L. Goeders, C. Kane, J. Briscoe, *Are Physicians Ready for MACRA/QPP? Results From a KPMG-AMA Survey*, Washington, D.C.: KPMG, 2017.

Krivich, R. S., "What Closings Mean to the Direct Primary Care Model: Two Prominent Direct Pay Practices Are Shutting Their Doors, Prompting Questions About the Movement's Future," *Medical Economics*, Vol. 94, No. 13, 2017, pp. 50–51.

Kuramoto, R. K., "Specialties: Missing in Our Healthcare Reform Strategies?" *Journal of Healthcare Management*, Vol. 59, No. 2, 2014, pp. 89–94.

Kvale, S., *Interviews: An Introduction to Qualitative Research Writing*, Thousand Oaks, Calif.: Sage Publications, 1996.

Leslie, B. M., and M. L. Blau, "Survival Strategies in a Changing Practice Environment," *Journal of Hand Surgery*, Vol. 39, No. 5, 2014, pp. 1012–1016.

Levine, D. M., J. A. Linder, and B. E. Landon, "Characteristics and Disparities Among Primary Care Practices in the United States," *Journal of General Internal Medicine*, Vol. 33, No. 4, 2018, pp. 481–486.

Lewis, V. A., K. Schoenherr, T. Fraze, and A. Cunningham, "Clinical Coordination in Accountable Care Organizations: A Qualitative Study," *Health Care Management Review*, December 6, 2016.

Lewis, V. A., K. I. Tierney, C. H. Colla, and S. M. Shortell, "The New Frontier of Strategic Alliances in Health Care: New Partnerships Under Accountable Care Organizations," *Social Science & Medicine*, Vol. 190, 2017, pp. 1–10.

Lieberman, J. R., R. M. Molloy, and B. D. Springer, "Practice Management Strategies Among Current Members of the American Association of Hip and Knee Surgeons," *Journal of Arthroplasty*, Vol. 33, No. 7s, 2018, pp. S19–S22.

Livingston, S., "No Appointment? No Problem . . . for a Price," *Modern Healthcare*, Vol. 47, No. 43, 2017, pp. 0024–0024.

Luder, H. R., P. Shannon, J. Kirby, and S. M. Frede, "Community Pharmacist Collaboration with a Patient-Centered Medical Home: Establishment of a Patient-Centered Medical Neighborhood and Payment Model," *Journal of the American Pharmaceutical Association*, Vol. 58, No. 1, 2018, pp. 44–50.

MacLean, C. H., E. A. Kerr, and A. Qaseem, "Time Out—Charting a Path for Improving Performance Measurement," *New England Journal of Medicine*, Vol. 378, No. 19, 2018, pp. 1757–1761.

Maeng, D. D., N. Khan, J. Tomcavage, T. R. Graf, D. E. Davis, and G. D. Steele, "Reduced Acute Inpatient Care Was Largest Savings Component of Geisinger Health System's Patient-Centered Medical Home," *Health Affairs (Millwood)*, Vol. 34, No. 4, 2015, pp. 636–644.

McHugh, J. P., A. Foster, V. Mor, R. R. Shield, A. N. Trivedi, T. Wetle, J. S. Zinn, and D. A. Tyler, "Reducing Hospital Readmissions Through Preferred Networks of Skilled Nursing Facilities," *Health Affairs*, Vol. 36, No. 9, 2017, pp. 1591–1598.

McWilliams, J. M., L. G. Gilstrap, D. G. Stevenson, M. E. Chernew, H. A. Huskamp, and D. C. Grabowski, "Changes in Postacute Care in the Medicare Shared Savings Program," *JAMA Internal Medicine*, Vol. 177, No. 4, 2017, pp. 518–526.

Mechanic, R. E., "Opportunities and Challenges for Payment Reform: Observations from Massachusetts," *Journal of Health Politics, Policy and Law*, Vol. 41, No. 4, 2016, pp. 743–762.

"Are Physicians Ready for Medicare Pay Reform?" *Medical Economics*, Vol. 94, No. 15, 2017. As of October 11, 2018:
http://search.ebscohost.com/login.aspx?direct=true&db=bth&AN=124285849&site=ehost-live

The Medicus Firm, "15th Annual Physician Practice Preference and Relocation Survey Released by The Medicus Firm," July 18, 2018. As of August 8, 2018:
https://www.themedicusfirm.com/news/15th-annual-physician-practice-preference-and-relocation-survey-released-by-the-medicus-firm

Meyer, H., "Bundled-Payment Joint Replacement Programs Winning Over Surgeons," *Modern Healthcare*, Vol. 47, No. 41, 2017. As of October 11, 2018:
http://www.modernhealthcare.com/article/20171007/NEWS/171009950

———, "Bundled Payment Success Varies by Condition," *Modern Healthcare*, Vol. 48, No. 5, 2018. As of October 11, 2018:
http://www.modernhealthcare.com/article/20180127/NEWS/180129938

Muchmore, S., "Few Docs Ready for Risk," *Modern Healthcare*, Vol. 46, No. 33, 2016, pp. 0020–0020.

Muldoon, L. D., P. M. Pelizzari, K. A. Lang, J. Vandigo, and B. S. Pyenson, "Assessing Medicare's Approach to Covering New Drugs in Bundled Payments for Oncology," *Health Affairs (Millwood)*, Vol. 37, No. 5, 2018, pp. 743–750.

Murciano-Goroff, Y. R., A. M. McCarthy, M. N. Bristol, S. M. Domchek, P. W. Groeneveld, U. N. Motanya, and K. Armstrong, "Medical Oncologists' Willingness to Participate in Bundled Payment Programs," *BMC Health Services Research*, Vol. 18, No. 1, 2018, p. 391.

Neprash, H. T., M. E. Chernew, and J. M. McWilliams, "Little Evidence Exists to Support the Expectation That Providers Would Consolidate to Enter New Payment Models," *Health Affairs (Millwood)*, Vol. 36, No. 2, 2017, pp. 346–354.

Okunogbe, A., L. S. Meredith, E. T. Chang, A. Simon, S. E. Stockdale, and L. V. Rubenstein, "Care Coordination and Provider Stress in Primary Care Management of High-Risk Patients," *Journal of General Internal Medicine*, Vol. 33, No. 1, 2018, pp. 65–71.

O'Malley, A. S., R. Sarwar, R. Keith, P. Balke, S. Ma, and N. McCall, "Provider Experiences with Chronic Care Management (CCM) Services and Fees: A Qualitative Research Study," *Journal of General Internal Medicine*, Vol. 32, No. 12, 2017, pp. 1294–1300.

Panjamapirom, T., and R. Lazerow, "10 Takeaways on the 2018 MACRA Final Rule," *At the Helm*, November 3, 2017. As of August 1, 2018:
https://www.advisory.com/research/health-care-advisory-board/blogs/at-the-helm/2017/11/2018-macra-final-rule

Peikes, D., S. Dale, A. Ghosh, E. F. Taylor, K. Swankoski, A. S. O'Malley, T. J. Day, N. Duda, P. Singh, G. Anglin, L. L. Sessums, and R. S. Brown, "The Comprehensive Primary Care Initiative: Effects on Spending, Quality, Patients, and Physicians," *Health Affairs (Millwood)*, Vol. 37, No. 6, 2018, pp. 890–899.

Perez, K., "Implications of Dartmouth-Hitchcock's Departure from the Pioneer ACO Program," *HFM (Healthcare Financial Management)*, Vol. 70, No. 1, 2016, p. 88.

Pines, J. M., P. Penninti, S. Alfaraj, J. N. Carlson, O. Colfer, C. K. Corbit, and A. Venkat, "Measurement Under the Microscope: High Variability and Limited Construct Validity in Emergency Department Patient-Experience Scores," *Annals of Emergency Medicine*, Vol. 71, No. 5, 2018, pp. 545–554, E546.

Pittman, P., and E. Forrest, "The Changing Roles of Registered Nurses in Pioneer Accountable Care Organizations," *Nursing Outlook*, Vol. 63, No. 5, 2015, pp. 554–565.

Pofeldt, E., "The Rise of Direct Primary Care," *Medical Economics*, Vol. 93, No. 7, 2016, pp. 42–46.

Prudencio, J., T. Cutler, S. Roberts, S. Marin, and M. Wilson, "The Effect of Clinical Pharmacist-Led Comprehensive Medication Management on Chronic Disease State Goal Attainment in a Patient-Centered Medical Home," *Journal of Managed Care & Specialty Pharmacy*, Vol. 24, No. 5, 2018, pp. 423–429.

Quinn, K., "Physician Payment Methods and the Patient-Centered Medical Home: Comment on 'A Troubled Asset Relief Program for the Patient-Centered Medical Home,'" *Journal of Ambulatory Care Management*, Vol. 40, No. 2, 2017, pp. 114–120.

Rama, A., *Payment and Delivery in 2016: The Prevalence of Medical Homes, Accountable Care Organizations, and Payment Methods Reported By Physicians*, Policy Research Perspectives, Washington, D.C.: American Medical Association, 2017.

Reindl, J., "Some GM Employees to Get 'Direct-to-Employer' Health Care Option," *Detroit Free Press*, August 6, 2018. As of September 20, 2018:
https://www.freep.com/story/money/2018/08/06/gm-direct-employer-health-insurance-2019/913210002/

Resnick, M. J., A. J. Graves, M. B. Buntin, M. R. Richards, and D. F. Penson, "Surgeon Participation in Early Accountable Care Organizations," *Annals of Surgery*, Vol. 267, No. 3, 2018, pp. 401–407.

Richards, M. R., C. T. Smith, A. J. Graves, M. B. Buntin, and M. J. Resnick, "Physician Competition in the Era of Accountable Care Organizations," *Health Services Research*, Vol. 53, No. 2, 2018, pp. 1272–1285.

Roberts, E. T., A. M. Zaslavsky, and J. M. McWilliams, "The Value-Based Payment Modifier: Program Outcomes and Implications for Disparities," *Annals of Internal Medicine*, Vol. 168, No. 4, 2018, pp. 255–265.

Rogers, E. A., S. T. Manser, J. Cleary, A. M. Joseph, E. M. Harwood, and K. T. Call, "Integrating Community Health Workers into Medical Homes," *Annals of Family Medicine*, Vol. 16, No. 1, 2018, pp. 14–20.

Sarinopoulos, I., D. L. Bechel-Marriott, J. M. Malouin, S. Zhai, J. C. Forney, and C. L. Tanner, "Patient Experience with the Patient-Centered Medical Home in Michigan's Statewide Multi-Payer Demonstration: A Cross-Sectional Study," *Journal of General Internal Medicine*, Vol. 32, No. 11, 2017, pp. 1202–1209.

Schulz, J., M. Decamp, and S. A. Berkowitz, "Medicare Shared Savings Program: Public Reporting and Shared Savings Distributions," *American Journal of Managed Care*, Vol. 21, No. 8, 2015, pp. 546–553.

Schur, C. L., and J. P. Sutton, "Physicians in Medicare ACOs Offer Mixed Views of Model for Health Care Cost and Quality," *Health Affairs (Millwood)*, Vol. 36, No. 4, 2017, pp. 649–654.

Shakir, M., K. Armstrong, and J. H. Wasfy, "Could Pay-for-Performance Worsen Health Disparities?" *Journal of General Internal Medicine*, Vol. 33, No. 4, 2018, pp. 567–569.

Shortell, S. M., S. R. McClellan, P. P. Ramsay, L. P. Casalino, A. M. Ryan, and K. R. Copeland, "Physician Practice Participation in Accountable Care Organizations: The Emergence of the Unicorn," *Health Services Research*, Vol. 49, No. 5, 2014, pp. 1519–1536.

Song, Z., S. Rose, D. G. Safran, B. E. Landon, M. P. Day, and M. E. Chernew, "Changes in Health Care Spending and Quality 4 Years into Global Payment," *New England Journal of Medicine*, Vol. 371, No. 18, 2014, pp. 1704–1714.

Stanowski, A. C., K. Simpson, and A. White, "Pay for Performance: Are Hospitals Becoming More Efficient in Improving Their Patient Experience?" *Journal of Healthcare Management*, Vol. 60, No. 4, 2015, pp. 268–285.

Stecker, E. C., "Why the Oregon CCO Experiment Could Founder," *Journal of Health Politics, Policy and Law*, Vol. 39, No. 4, 2014, pp. 941–946.

Stock, R., J. Hall, A. M. Chang, and D. Cohen, "Physicians' Early Perspectives on Oregon's Coordinated Care Organizations," *Healthcare (Amst)*, Vol. 4, No. 2, 2016, pp. 92–97.

Takach, M., C. Townley, R. Yalowich, and S. Kinsler, "Making Multipayer Reform Work: What Can Be Learned from Medical Home Initiatives," *Health Affairs (Millwood)*, Vol. 34, No. 4, 2015, pp. 662–672.

Tejedor-Sojo, J., T. Creek, and T. Leong, "Impact of Audit and Feedback and Pay-for-Performance Interventions on Pediatric Hospitalist Discharge Communication with Primary Care Providers," *American Journal of Medical Quality*, Vol. 30, No. 2, 2015, pp. 149–155.

Terry, K. E. N., "Reporting Quality Data Through an ACO: Value-Based Pay Adds to Physicians' Paperwork Burdens, But the Right Accountable Care Organizations Can Help," *Medical Economics*, Vol. 95, No. 1, 2018, pp. 23–26.

Tsai, T. C., K. E. Joynt, R. C. Wild, E. J. Orav, and A. K. Jha, "Medicare's Bundled Payment Initiative: Most Hospitals Are Focused on a Few High-Volume Conditions," *Health Affairs (Millwood)*, Vol. 34, No. 3, 2015, pp. 371–380.

Urdapilleta, O., D. Weinberg, S. Pedersen, G. Kim, S. Cannon-Jones, and J. Woodward, *Evaluation of the Medicare Acute Care Episode (ACE) Demonstration: Final Evaluation Report*, Impaq International, 2013. As of October 11, 2018:
https://downloads.cms.gov/files/cmmi/ACE-EvaluationReport-Final-5-2-14.pdf

Van Dyke, M., "Ready Set Go! Rural Hospitals Have a Lot to Watch for as the New Medicare Quality Payment Program Kicks In (Cover Story)," *Trustee*, Vol. 70, No. 1, 2017, pp. 8–12.

Vaughn, T., A. C. MacKinney, K. J. Mueller, F. Ullrich, and X. Zhu, "Medicare Accountable Care Organizations: Beneficiary Assignment Update," *Rural Policy Brief*, Vol. 2, 2016, pp. 1–7.

Wadhera, R. K., R. W. Yeh, and K. E. Joynt Maddox, "The Rise and Fall of Mandatory Cardiac Bundled Payments," *JAMA*, Vol. 319, No. 4, 2018, pp. 335–336.

Wagner, E. H., M. Flinter, C. Hsu, D. Cromp, B. T. Austin, R. Etz, B. F. Crabtree, and M. D. Ladden, "Effective Team-Based Primary Care: Observations from Innovative Practices," *BMC Family Practice*, Vol. 18, No. 1, 2017, p. 13.

Walker, T., "Specialty Intensive Medical Home," *Managed Healthcare Executive*, Vol. 27, No. 4, 2017, pp. 30–31.

Wan, S., P. G. Teichman, D. Latif, J. Boyd, and R. Gupta, "Healthcare Provider Perceptions of the Role of Interprofessional Care in Access to and Outcomes of Primary Care in an Underserved Area," *Journal of Interprofessional Care*, Vol. 32, No. 2, 2018, pp. 220–223.

Wasfy, J. H., C. M. Zigler, C. Choirat, Y. Wang, F. Dominici, and R. W. Yeh, "Readmission Rates After Passage of the Hospital Readmissions Reduction Program: A Pre-Post Analysis," *Annals of Internal Medicine*, Vol. 166, No. 5, 2017, pp. 324–331.

Wax, C. M., "Physician Accountability? Let's Legislate Congressional Accountability," *Medical Economics*, Vol. 94, No. 21, 2017, p. 8.

Whitcomb, W. F., T. Lagu, R. J. Krushell, A. P. Lehman, J. Greenbaum, J. McGirr, P. S. Pekow, S. Calcasola, E. Benjamin, J. Mayforth, and P. K. Lindenauer, "Experience with Designing and Implementing a Bundled Payment Program for Total Hip Replacement," *Joint Commission Journal on Quality and Patient Safety*, Vol. 41, No. 9, 2015, pp. 406–413.

Whitman, E., "Delivering New Bundles to Control Cost of Maternal Care," *Modern Healthcare*, Vol. 46, No. 33, 2016a. As of October 11, 2018:
https://www.pressreader.com/usa/modern-healthcare/20160815/281668254373376

———, "Rapid Adoption of Bundled Payments Remains an Act of Faith," *Modern Healthcare*, Vol. 46, No. 39, 2016b, p. 14.

———, "Will Value-Based Payment Initiatives Continue Under Trump?" *Modern Healthcare*, Vol. 46, No. 46, 2016c, p. 0018.

Wiley, J. A., D. R. Rittenhouse, S. M. Shortell, L. P. Casalino, P. P. Ramsay, S. Bibi, A. M. Ryan, K. R. Copeland, and J. A. Alexander, "Managing Chronic Illness: Physician Practices Increased the Use of Care Management and Medical Home Processes," *Health Affairs (Millwood)*, Vol. 34, No. 1, 2015, pp. 78–86.

Wise, C. G., J. A. Alexander, L. A. Green, and G. R. Cohen, "Physician Organization-Practice Team Integration for the Advancement of Patient-Centered Care," *Journal of Ambulatory Care Management*, Vol. 35, No. 4, 2012, pp. 311–322.

Wolinsky, H., "With MACRA Looming, Doctors Can't Afford Waiting to Plumb Its Intricacies," *Modern Healthcare*, Vol. 46, No. 29, 2016. As of October 11, 2018:
http://www.modernhealthcare.com/article/20160723/MAGAZINE/307239981

Xu, Y., and P. S. Wells, "Getting (Along) with the Guidelines: Reconciling Patient Autonomy and Quality Improvement Through Shared Decision Making," *Academic Medicine*, Vol. 91, No. 7, 2016, pp. 925–929.

Yin, R. K., *Case Study Research: Design and Methods*, Thousand Oaks, Calif.: Sage Publications, 2014.

Young, A., H. J. Chaudhry, X. Pei, K. Arnhart, M. Dugan, and G. B. Snyder, "A Census of Actively Licensed Physicians in the United States, 2016," *Journal of Medical Regulation*, Vol. 103, No. 2, 2017, pp. 7–21.

Zuvekas, S. H., and J. W. Cohen, "Fee-for-Service, While Much Maligned, Remains the Dominant Payment Method for Physician Visits," *Health Affairs (Millwood)*, Vol. 35, No. 3, 2016, pp. 411–414.

Zygourakis, C. C., V. Valencia, C. Moriates, C. K. Boscardin, S. Catschegn, A. Rajkomar, K. J. Bozic, K. Soo Hoo, A. N. Goldberg, L. Pitts, M. T. Lawton, R. A. Dudley, and R. Gonzales, "Association Between Surgeon Scorecard Use and Operating Room Costs," *JAMA Surgery*, Vol. 152, No. 3, 2017, pp. 284–291.

Made in the USA
Middletown, DE
25 April 2021

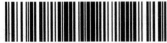